TheraQi

*Move Your Way to
Happiness and Health*

Jason Rockwood
TheraQi LLC

Jason Rockwood
TheraQi LLC
123 S.E. 3rd Avenue, Suite 372
Miami, FL 33131
www.theraqi.com

TheraQi is a Trademark of TheraQi LLC

Publisher's Note: This book is for educational purposes. The publisher and author of this instructional book are not responsible in any manner whatsoever for any adverse effects arising directly or indirectly as a result of the information provided in this book. If not practiced safely and with caution, any workout out can be dangerous to you and to others. It is highly recommended to consult with a professional fitness instructor before beginning training. It is also very important to consult with a physician prior to training due to the intense and strenuous nature of the techniques in this book. Neither Jason Rockwood nor TheraQi LLC shall be liable or responsible for any loss or damage allegedly arising from any information or suggestion in this book.

TheraQi / Jason Rockwood. — 1st ed.

ISBN-13: 978-0692869062 (TheraQi LLC)

ISBN-10: 0692869069

Acknowledgements

I wish to acknowledge all the wonderful friends in my life who have supported me over the years as I've worked to bring this book to reality. Thanks to my mother, Sheila, for being my first student. Thank you to Jennifer Iannolo, who validated the difference this workout can make. Thank you to my dear friend Stephen Dolginoff, who was the first person to tell me to "write it down," and wisely counseled me to "never let the perfect be the enemy of the good." Thank you to Kim Kostus, who provided the inspiration and the magic. Thanks to Leslee Drogowitz for her eagle eye. A huge thanks to Gary Montalvo for his design expertise and generosity. I have eternal gratitude to Harvey Helms for blazing a trail for us both. Much love to Kino, who provided the foundation. And finally, a very special thank you to Dev Ramnarine, who makes miracles happen every day both physical and metaphysical.

I love you all.

Jason

To my family and friends.

"WHEN BIRTHING A NEW REALITY,
DANCING WITH CHAOS IS NECESSARY."

-Dev Ramnarine

Table of Contents

The Story of TheraQi

How this book and method came to life.

I have a confession. I don't like working out. I never did. I always hated it. Lifting weights hurt my body and made me sore. Running was exhausting and hard on my knees. Aerobics made me short of breath. Yoga hurt like hell and was beyond boring. I was convinced that I would never have a good body or be physically fit.

Then, in 2003, I spent a year living in Moscow, Russia. Through a strange turn of events, I became friends with a group of men who worked for the Russian Secret Service. These guys were tough. They had beautiful, sculpted, strong bodies and could perform unimaginable feats of strength. When I asked them their secret to staying fit, they explained (in their heavy Russian accent) that "to have a strong body, you must do one of two things: lift the weights, or do the movements."

"Do the movements?" I asked. What did that mean? It sounded intriguing. Any alternative to lifting weights sounded good to me!

My Russian friends then started teaching me their method for exercising: a series of innocuous (and even silly-looking) movements that proved to be deceptively simple but powerful. The movements looked easy, and could be, but could also become quite challenging when performed intentionally and repeatedly. Some of the movements reminded me of ballet, another Russian method which I had previously studied. And while the movements were dynamic, rather than static poses, the feeling of stretching and opening the body reminded me a little of yoga.

What I found was that these movements were fiercely effective at strengthening and toning my body. Best of all, they were fun. They felt good. When I was finished working out, I had more energy than when I began. I felt oddly relaxed and energized at the same time. And over time, I lost weight, gained muscle, and improved my fitness on nearly every metric possible.

When I returned to the US, I began doing research and discovered that the training I received was called Systema. Systema is a little-known Russian martial art based on traditional Russian and Cossack sword-fighting and dancing techniques. Cossack dancing, much like Brazilian Capoeira or Hawaiian Hula dancing, is a form of martial art training. Warriors in these different cultures were chosen based on their ability to dance. Under Communism, Stalin refined the Systema fighting method for use by the KGB and other elite fighters, while prohibiting anyone outside the military to study the method. After the fall of the Soviet Union, the practice of Systema began to leak out in a trickle. Today, knowledge of Systema is limited to only a few martial arts specialists in Russia, and remains little-known outside of that country.

I want to make clear I'm not a martial artist. Not at all. Systema is a technique for fighting, and I wasn't interested in that. I was interested in the way it supported my health and wellbeing. The philosophy behind Systema was very Eastern in its mindset. It was holistic, mental as well as physical, and designed to stimulate health. The term "system" in Systema refers to how the method stimulates and strengthens the 11 systems of bodily health: cardiovascular, pulmonary, reproductive, endocrine, skin, muscle, skeletal, lymphatic, digestive, urinary, and nervous systems. Over time, I found myself experiencing a range of mental and physical improvements that traditional exercise had never provided me. I was fascinated by the benefits I experienced from these movements and decided to find out more.

I began to research related fields about joint movement, and began to make more sense of what I was doing, and why it worked the miracles I experienced.

I stumbled upon a movement approach called "neurodynamics", a combination of overlapping but related areas in osteopathy/chiropractics, physical therapy, and injury rehabilitation. This psycho-social approach to the body and how it moves merges joint movements with intense mental focus to produce higher levels of bodily control and function. It gets very geeky and academic, but proponents argue that it helps with rehabilitating injuries, reducing pain, and giving athletes higher levels of physical performance. Many of the exercises, or "dynamic joint mobilizations" are movements that were familiar to me as part of my Russian training. One neurodynamic training company had a name, "Z-Health", that was even based on a Russian word meaning health: "Z'darovyeh." It seemed like neurodynamic joint mobilizations were the Western academic equivalent of my Eastern martial art tradition.

At the same time I was doing this research, I began spending time on the Caribbean island of St.

Barts. It was the first time in my life I actively took up swimming. I went to the beach at least once if not twice a day. I felt amazing. Swimming is truly a magical form of exercise. If only everyone had access to the beach!

When I came back to New York City, it became impractical to swim every day. How, I asked myself, could I keep the benefits of swimming without needing the water? I realized that the joint movements I was practicing all these years from Systema were very similar to swimming, and I began to formulate a sequence of movements I could practice every day, a sequence that would leave me feeling as energized and refreshed as if I had gone for a swim in the ocean.

I loved the workout I was developing and I wanted to share it. Trying to explain it to people turned out to be a struggle. "Swimming on land?" "Russian what?" "Neuro-who?" Their confusion was understandable. I wasn't even certain how to describe it. Was it cardio, or strength training? (Both, but neither.) Was it yoga? (No, but kind of.) Was it dance? (Not really, but sort of.)

Despite the confusion about what it was, I was crystal clear about the benefits it provided. People who did my workout spoke of decreased pain, increased mobility, and overall improvement in well-being—the same benefits predicted by the physiologists writing about neurodynamics.

Then in 2014, over 10 years since I had first started developing this program, I traveled to Hong Kong. As I wandered the streets of Kowloon, I saw many older Chinese people doing workouts in the streets, workouts that looked surprisingly similar to my Russian-inspired routine. I found out they were practicing QiGong. QiGong literally means "life energy cultivation" and is a practice of aligning body, breath, and mind for health, meditation, and martial arts training. This was the closest thing I had found to describing my workout: a practice using gentle, energy stimulating movements to produce health, clarity, and fitness.

Qi is an important concept present in many Eastern movement traditions. The Japanese have "Ki" (like in Aikido or Reiki), the Chinese have "Qi" (like in QiGong), and the yoga tradition has "prana". Western fitness traditions completely leave this concept out, perhaps because it is not scientifically proven to exist. Nevertheless, I believe that Qi, or "bio-energy", is the source of why these Eastern movement methods are such powerful contributors to health and happiness. Qi-based exercises are both energizing and relaxing at the same time. Qi-focused activity calms the mind and invigorates the body. I liked the idea of including Qi in my workout philosophy and sharing this concept with my American friends. My method was not pure QiGong or Systema or any other existing method. Tai chi, QiGong, and other martial arts practices require a high level of focus and mental and physical discipline. These disciplines weren't practical for sharing with a wide audience. I was determined to bring this amazing method of movement to people who typically didn't exercise, such as those with chronic pain, obesity, advanced age, or those recovering from illness. My approach was more therapeutic than it was about getting fit or achieving mastery. It was clear that while my method was similar to, and inspired by, these other practices, it was unique enough to share distinctly.

I chose to call my method TheraQi, taken from the Greek word for healing and the Chinese word for energy. "Healing Energy" was exactly the concept I had in mind that I wanted to share with the people in my life who I knew would benefit tremendously from this method.

TheraQi is inspired by yoga, Systema, swimming, dynamic joint mobility exercises, ballet, QiGong, and other forms of dance. Each of these practices in and of itself offers a fantastic mode of physical health, and if you have the available time, energy, and resources, I wholly encourage you to practice them! The problem is that these methods of exercise are not universally accessible. Swimming requires a source of water. Systema, QiGong, yoga and ballet all require a level of discipline and commitment that makes them impractical for the general population. A majority of the people who could benefit from these forms of exercise never will. People either won't be exposed to them or won't be able to "keep up" even if they tried. These specialized fitness methods require specialized instruction and a very focused, dedicated practice. The end result is that people get left behind, and an otherwise beneficial movement method goes untried.

I am passionate about the TheraQi method because I believe it is truly a universal fitness program. I have done this workout with overweight people, the elderly, and people with fibromyalgia. I've also done it with professional athletes, jujitsu champions, and doctors. Everyone I do the workout with reports feeling better when they finished than when they began. Each person reports a unique experience and set of benefits, even though the sequence is universally the same. People who do it regularly report weight loss, increased athletic performance, pain reduction, increased flexibility, and an improved sense of mood and well-being. Some people even report it helps them sleep more soundly. TheraQi offers the maximum benefit for the least investment. It's the smartest exercise program you will ever encounter. And best of all, anyone can do it.

No matter what your fitness level, I invite you to try TheraQi and see for yourself what is possible. You will be surprised what you learn about your body and how you move it. Best of all, you'll be surprised at how good exercise can make you feel. That makes TheraQi its own reward.

What is TheraQi?

Circumduction, what's your function?

TheraQi is a low-impact yoga-alternative that's easy, energizing, and enjoyable.

The sequence of movements in the TheraQi method is uniquely my own, but the individual movements in TheraQi are not. This is part of why the movements are valuable—I didn't just make them up, they have been proven by others in many diverse fields. The problem is that these movements have historically been spread out across many disciplines, some of which are very specialized. They are not accessible in any coherent method. TheraQi is my personal synthesis of what I consider to be the most beneficial movements for stimulating happiness and health, presented in a cohesive, accessible system.

Just as no one "owns" the movements of yoga, no one owns the movements in TheraQi. What this book does is present movements to you that are unfamiliar, or present familiar movements to you in a new way. I have attempted, for each movement in the TheraQi sequence, to associate the movement to something familiar and recognizable, whether from the gym, from dance, or from yoga.

A key element of what makes the movements in TheraQi effective and unique is that they are based on circular movements instead of linear ones. Lifting a dumbbell up and down is a linear movement. Swinging a tennis racket or a golf club is a circular movement. Circular movements play a minor role in mainstream fitness, and a major role in TheraQi. That's what makes TheraQi different from other methods of exercise. Circular movements have many benefits. By the time you finish this book, you will understand those benefits for yourself.

There are two types of circles that play a special role in TheraQi.

The first is a "hula" motion. Hula motion is a circular/sliding motion of the vertebrae in the spine. Broadly, you can "hula" your pelvis, hips, chest, or head. Each of these areas can be moved in a circle isolated from the rest of the body. These hula motions expand the range of motion in the spine, making it supple and flexible. At the same time, hula motions stimulate the nervous system and other bodily systems.

The second special circular motion is called circumduction. Circumduction plays a very critical role in TheraQi. Most forms of traditional exercise focus on "flexing" and "extending." When you pull a weight towards you (like a bicep curl) you are flexing. When you push weight away from your body (like in a bench press) you are extending. But there's another way of moving we rarely think about: moving weight (or a body part) in a circle. Circumduction is defined as the circular movement of any part of the body that is attached at one end and open on the other. A hand can circumduct at the wrist; the eyes circumduct in their sockets; a foot can circumduct at the ankle; the leg circumducts at the hip, etc. If you make an arm circle like you're swimming, that's circumduction. Circumduction is a powerful motion that combines flexing and extending across 360 degrees. Circumduction expands range of motion, stimulates the nervous system, lubricates the joints, and strengthens both major and minor muscle groups.

If the TheraQi method could be summed up in one phrase, it would be "Circumduct every major joint, every single day."

Circumduction, and circular movement in general, are not well-taught in Western physical education. I believe that this is because circumduction is both too easy and too hard for most people. On the one hand, it's very easy to twirl your arm around in a big circle. It may seem at first glance like nothing is happening (though do it 50 times and see how you feel). On the other hand, circumduction is difficult. You may be able to bicep curl a 20 pound weight, but if you try and circumduct it from the elbow or shoulder, you may find that you are only able to lift 5 pounds. This is because circumduction shifts the center of gravity of weight, making the weight harder to lift. Circumduction doesn't activate the major muscle groups as much the supporting, stabilizing muscles near the joints and the core. This makes circumduction ideal for building strength but bad for building mass. Circumduction will make your body lean, strong, and flexible, but it won't make you "swole." Perhaps that's why this magical motion plays second fiddle in our "bigger is better" culture. Focusing on large (read: eye-catching) muscle groups while ignoring the joints and minor muscle groups means we lose out on the health benefits of stimulating the 11 systems of the body. I prefer to focus on the holistic benefits of motion, rather than building mass or reducing fat. Movement, not muscle, is the key to happiness and health.

When we break free of the obsession with low-fat, high-muscle bodies, we discover the intrinsic pleasure in movement. Like dance, movement is its own reward. It feels good, it's simple, and it's fun. The requirements to participate in strenuous programs like yoga, running, or weightlifting prevent many people from participating. TheraQi, however, is perfect for anyone, because people's bodies are perfect just the way they are. There's nothing to fix or change. When we love our bodies and how they move, movement becomes a natural form of self expression. We burn fat and build muscle as a byproduct of our love of motion, not as an end in itself. Exercise becomes something we want to do, not something we have to do. TheraQi is a way out of the endless cycle of guilt, over-exertion, burnout, and more guilt. With TheraQi, you'll find yourself craving movement, not avoiding it. No matter what, you will discover your body is perfect. You are always ready to move, in any conditions, in any circumstances, regardless of age, body type, or physical ability.

My approach to fitness sounds revolutionary compared to the endless parade of high-intensity, pain-inducing fitness programs peddled in the West, but my approach to movement is not so foreign in many Asian traditions.

In Japan, there is something called *rajio taiso*, which means "radio exercises" or "radio stretches." Every morning on the national Japanese radio channel at 6:30 AM, you can hear the instructions for doing the morning stretch routine, which has been broadcast daily, virtually unchanged, since the 1930's. Much like TheraQi, *rajio taiso* features lots of arm circles, bends, squats, and toe touches. Almost every school in Japan uses *rajio taiso* to help students warm up before sports and physical education classes. Japanese corporations use *rajio taiso* to keep employees healthy and build morale. Japan has many martial and healing arts which reference Qi (the Japanese pronounce it "Ki"), such as reiki ("soul-energy") and aikido ("the way of unifying the life energy").

In China, you can find elderly ladies and gentlemen doing QiGong in the alley ways and public parks, just as naturally as going for a walk. They don't have any sense of embarrassment or shame about exercising in public. On the contrary, it's very beautiful to watch. It's not uncommon to see workers stop in the middle of what they are doing to take a quick rest to stretch, twist, bend over, and flap their arms like a bird. QiGong also stimulates the body through circular movement.

Eastern cultures (including Russia, which borders China) have a special relationship to gentle, stimulating exercise, which they undertake daily for health, longevity, and well-being. Contrast this to the American approach to fitness, which is obsessed with being stronger, faster, bigger, smaller, etc. The American style of exercise can be exhausting, boring, painful, and sometimes dangerous. The old ladies doing QiGong aren't trying to get washboard abs, they just want to feel good and live a long life.

Just like with *rajio taiso*, TheraQi is intended to be performed every morning, every day, for pretty much the rest of your life. Just like you eat every day, you sleep every day, you do lots of things every day, because health is something that requires daily maintenance. TheraQi is meant to be part of your morning wakeup routine. Consider it the extra twenty minutes you're going to put into your morning along with your coffee and shower to start your day off right. It's not going to give you the body of a champion bodybuilder, but you'll soon discover it's a wonderful way to wake up your body, mind, and spirit. If it gives you the energy to do more, great, but if it's all you do, you'll be better off for it.

There's an additional, important benefit to a daily TheraQi practice that comes from doing the same movements every day. When practiced daily, the TheraQi sequence becomes a diagnostic tool, a barometer for your overall health. Going through the various movements in the sequence, day after day, you begin to get familiar with your body at a level that you probably never imagined. You discover your body like getting to know an old friend. You learn where you have pain, where you get stuck, where you find yourself struggling. If you wake up one morning and discover that the routine is taking more effort than usual, or if a usually comfortable movement suddenly feels painful, that's valuable information for understanding your overall state of health. By the end of a TheraQi sequence, you will know what kind of condition your body is in and what it's going to take to get you through your day. Plan accordingly!

I passionately believe that Eastern-style "healing energy" exercise is the missing ingredient in Western health. We are endlessly told that the answer to our sedentary ways is more time on the treadmill, in the gym, or on the basketball court. It's not working. Our citizens are tired, overweight, and stressed out. Yoga, cardio, weightlifting, and athletics have a range of benefits, but most people do not have the energy and range of motion needed to fully participate. TheraQi is intended to bring the benefits of the Eastern-style morning movement program to the Western audience, without coming across as condescending, precious, complicated, or elitist.

I wrote this book for my family and friends, to give them access to a daily sequence of gentle movements for energy and health. I'm committed that we see energy movement and daily gentle exercise as a pleasurable, life affirming activity that brings joy and eliminates pain. And if that everyday practice of gentle movements empowers you to go on and lift weights or run, all the better. Lifting weights and running isn't necessary for health and wellness. TheraQi is. Doing it every day will change your life in ways you can't imagine, and once you start, you'll never go without it again. It feels that good, and I can't wait for you to begin.

Getting Started

*Practical considerations for getting
the most from a TheraQi practice.*

I like to do my morning movement sequence on a hard surface, such as a tiled floor or hardwood floor. Short carpet is also fine. You can perform TheraQi movements in any conditions. Don't worry if you have shag carpet on the floor. You can do the sequence lying in bed or sitting on the sofa if you like. Don't let the recommendations I make here dictate what you do. They are here as guidelines, not hard rules.

...

I like to do my workout with a large full body mirror or mirror wall. This way I can watch how my body moves and get a better understanding of my range of motion.

...

When doing the motions, never go beyond your comfort level. Adjust the movement to your body, your range of motion, your energy levels, etc. This is not a competition. Some of the movements can put strain on the joints, especially the knees. Trying to drop too low too fast, or overextending the spine, can cause serious injury. Always listen to your body to determine what's right for you.

...

I can't stress enough how important it is for you to do the workout your way.

...

Unlike similar methods like yoga or tai chi, the TheraQi method doesn't require you to breathe a certain way, "clear your mind" or move in a highly controlled, intentional manner. Life can be hectic, and sometimes it's hard to quiet the mind or concentrate on your breath. Sometimes just getting through the movement is enough. It's not that intentional movement and breath work are wrong, just that they aren't essential. You don't need to be a Zen master to do TheraQi. Come as you are.

...

TheraQi exercises depend a lot on the open movement of the feet. I therefore want to take a moment to address the various options for footwear.

Tennis shoes or sneakers are common exercise shoes, but sneakers don't provide a stable foundation for this workout. The thick soles prevent your feet from getting a firm grip on the ground. More importantly, sneakers prevent you from experiencing all your toes individually, and limit the range of motion for the ankle.

For this reason, you may want to do your TheraQi practice in either bare feet or socks. Some people, myself included, don't like being barefoot. Additionally, some movements require shifting weight onto the heels or balls of the feet, and that can irritate sensitive, delicate skin. If you are often barefoot and/or comfortable with it, doing the workout barefoot is fine. Barefoot on a yoga mat is also an option, though one I've never had good results with. The mat often bunches up under my feet or shifts around.

There's an alternative to going barefoot to consider. If you have the extra money available, I highly recommend purchasing a pair of "minimal shoes." These shoes are sometimes called "toe-shoes", because they are little more than pieces of rubber that slip on the feet. They have five individual spaces for each toe, which means that the foot gets the traction that comes from the rubber sole, but still allowing the toes to move independently. I love wearing these toe-shoes because they conform closely to the foot, protect it, and provide some traction to keep the foot grounded when doing other motions. Minimal toe-shoes provide my feet with the flexibility of being barefoot, but the protection of a shoe. While not necessary, I think they are well worth the investment, and will support you in getting the most out of your TheraQi practice.

...

The sequence is comprised of 50 movements that are divided into five sections: the core, the arms, the legs, the face, and compounds. Movements 1 to 21 are for the core: the spine, back, neck, belly, head, chest and clavicle. Movements 22 to 35 are for the arms: the fingers, hands, wrists, elbows and shoulders. Movements 36 to 43 are for the legs: the feet, ankles, knees and hips. Movements 44 and 45 are for the face and eyes. Movements 46, 47, 48 and 49 are compound movements that work various major muscle groups at the same time and provide a higher-intensity experience than the rest of the sequence. Movement 50 is a resting movement that should be executed at the end of every workout.

It's highly recommended to work through all fifty movements in the order presented, every single day. First thing in the morning is recommended. Once you learn the movements, this can easily be done in 30 minutes or less. If you're short on time, pick a few movements from each section (Core, Arms, Legs, Face, Compounds) always beginning with Figure 8 (Movement 1) and ending with Backbending (Movement 50).

•••

It's recommended that you spend the following amounts of time doing a TheraQi routine:

• 10 minutes if you're absolutely in a hurry;

• 20-30 minutes for maintaining daily health;

• 50-60 minutes to build and maintain a higher level of physical fitness;

• 70-90 minutes to burn fat and/or build muscle.

•••

I advise you to perform a complete TheraQi sequence every morning upon waking, and an abbreviated sequence before performing any physical activity such as yoga, cardio, weightlifting, or athletics.

•••

In the beginning, you may struggle with some of the complex core movements or the vigorous compounds. Don't let this slow you down or prevent you from achieving your daily time goals. Focus on the Level 1 movements in the beginning; this will keep you moving until you master the more complex motions. The Levels of complexity are provided so that you can easily make a Level 1 routine for yourself and not get hung up on complexity or other challenge.

•••

While every attempt has been made to make this book a complete instruction manual, some moves may be easier to learn under the guidance of an instructor. Also, group classes are fun and the social aspect is motivating for many people. Working with an instructor one-on-one or in a group class is an excellent way to deepen your understanding of the TheraQi method.

•••

Whatever obstacles stand in your way, do the sequence anyway. If you're blind, have someone read to you or listen to a video. If you're confined to a bed, try to do what movements you can while lying down. If you're on a 24 hour flight to Asia, workout from your seat or in the bathroom. TheraQi is intended to be a universal workout for all ages, body types, and fitness levels. You can do TheraQi in any circumstances or conditions. Nothing can stop you from getting the benefits you desire, so get going, and get them every day no matter what.

1. FIGURE 8

*Move the hips in a horizontal figure
eight pattern parallel to the floor.*

Always begin your TheraQi routine by waking the lower core: the pelvis, hips, lower abdominals, lower back and butt. I highly recommend that you start your daily practice with the Figure 8, and only then move on to other movements in your routine. The Figure 8 provides an entire full-body warm-up that not only sets the stage for the rest of the sequence, it sets the stage for a healthy, happy day. It stimulates the digestive system and loosens tension in the hips and lower back, preparing you for whatever adventures await.

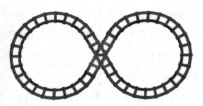 What is the Figure 8? Figure 8 is a way to execute a figure eight shape by moving the hips horizontally, parallel to the floor. First one hip describes half of the "8", and then the other hip describes the other half. The effect is that the pelvis traces out a figure eight shape around the body. It looks kind of like an infinity sign.

The Figure 8 motion can be either from front to back (a Backward Figure 8) or from back to front (a Forward Figure 8). I place more emphasis on the Forward Figure 8, but both are good to know and practice.

Figure 8 is a move very popular in Belly dancing, Hula, and Latin dance. In Latin dance, it's called "Latin Motion" or "Cuban Motion", and it's the foundation of dances such as merengue, salsa, rhumba, etc. Depending on the specific dance type, the Figure 8 in each of these dance traditions will look a little different, but the basic motion is universal. In TheraQi, I advise students to exaggerate the movement far more than in formal dance. The important thing is to make the movement your own and don't worry about the details.

Figure 8 is not physically demanding, but it does require coordination. The movement is easier to do when moving slowly and can become more vigorous as the music speeds up.

Figure 8 uses nearly every body part from the neck down. It works all the joints and many major muscles which is why it's important. Figure 8 is the first movement you'll learn and the last movement you'll master.

Once you get the hang of this wonderful horizontal figure eight motion, the other movements in the sequence will come quite easily.

Sometimes the instructions in this book will refer to the hips, and other times the pelvis. For our purposes, the pelvis refers to the entire structure of the lower body between the abdomen and the thighs, the "lower core." The general outer regions of the pelvis are called the hips, and the hip joints are where the thigh bones connect to the pelvis. In TheraQi, the hips or hip joints are often used to point in a specific direction or to trace a certain pattern in space. The pelvis is most often used to align the body in a particular manner. The two work together, since the best way to align the pelvis is to point the hip in a specific direction.

Figure 8 is one of the most complex movements in the sequence. It's also one of the most important. I take a long time to explain this single movement because there are many different nuances to discover about movement, about your body, and about your joints. I encourage you to patiently work through this chapter even if the movement comes to you naturally. The other movements in the sequence do not take as long to explain. On the other side, if you find this movement too complex, don't get discouraged from advancing to further chapters.

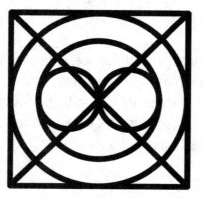

The TheraQi Movement Map

When I first started teaching a friend how to do Figure 8, she struggled to understand the hip motion I was describing. To make it easier for her to visualize the complex set of circles and angles that comprise this movement, I created a "TheraQi Movement Map." You may find this Movement Map helpful to learn how to move the hips, pelvis, and knees when doing the Figure 8 and many of the Hula movements in the Core section of the sequence.

If you have a good imagination, you can visualize the Movement Map on the floor underneath you. If you prefer, use a piece of chalk to draw it out on the sidewalk or the floor of your garage.

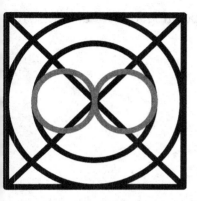

In the middle of the map are two small circles. Place your feet inside the two circles. These two circles are also used to trace the motion of the knees.

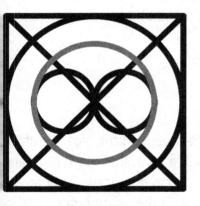

Next is the center circle. The center circle is used for making small Hula circles with the pelvis, particularly in Movement 16.

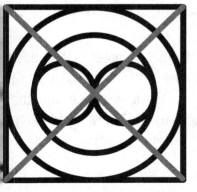

The X part of the map is used to align the pelvis. In the middle of a figure eight, there's a kind of x-shape. This X represents the two positions of the pelvis.

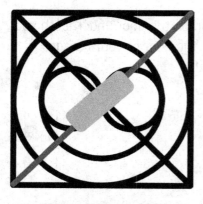

Position 1 is when the right hip is pointing forward and the left hip pointing back.

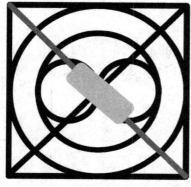

Position 2 is when the pelvis is pointed the other direction, with the left hip pointing forward and the right hip pointing back.

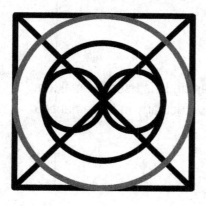

The outer circle is used to trace the motion of the hips. It's divided into four segments by the X, with a quarter in front, back and on each side. In Figure 8, only half the circle is used: the quarters on each side. In Hip Hula (Movement 17) the entire outer circle is used to guide the motion of the hips.

In addition to the use of the Movement Map, I like to break this somewhat complex motion down into three different levels to make it easier to learn. This gives everyone in the class the ability to follow along regardless of their level. I advise students to start with a pelvic twist (Level 1), then execute a Figure 8 with the hips (Level 2), and end by adding the knees to the Figure 8 and tying it all together (Level 3). By the time you've learned all three levels of the Figure 8, you'll have all the coordination you need to look good on the dance floor.

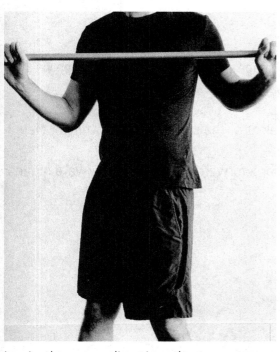

Level One: The Twist

Knowing how to isolate and twist the pelvis is key to the entire TheraQi sequence. Spend the first few days learning to move the pelvis before moving on to the other levels of the Figure 8.

Step 1: Begin in Starting Position, with feet shoulder width apart. Take a broom or other long handle and hold it close to the shoulders. This will help you see the position of your body more clearly.

Step 2: Keeping the feet firmly planted, rotate your upper body to face the upper left corner of the Movement Map, so that your pelvis is in line with Position 1. Both the shoulders and the hips are moving in the same direction; the torso turns as a single stable unit. Note that it's counterintuitive that by turning to the left, the pelvis points to the right.

Step 2: Rotate your upper body towards the upper right corner of the map, keeping the shoulders in line with the pelvis. This will move your pelvis into Position 2.

Step 3: Repeat this motion several times and come back to Starting Position to rest.

Step 4: Now isolate the pelvis from the upper torso. Hold the shoulders in Starting Position. Keeping the shoulders and head facing forward and the broom handle straight across the chest, isolate and rotate the pelvis back and forth between Position 1 and Position 2, while keeping the upper body still.

Step 6: Repeat this motion several times and come back to Starting Position to rest.

Level 2: The Horizontal Figure 8

At this level we use the hips to trace a figure eight shape in the space around the pelvis. The Movement Map illustrates the movement of the pelvis.

To ground the motion, picture in your mind the figure eight at the center of the Movement Map.

Trace the figure eight shape by moving the hips in either a forward motion or a backward motion.

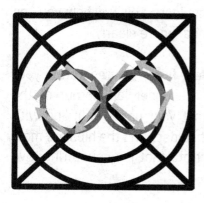

Moving forward from back to front.

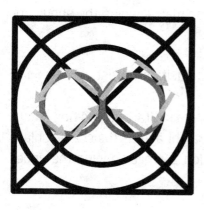

Moving backward from front to back.

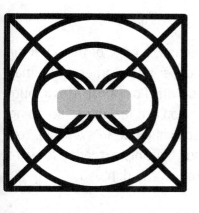

Forward Figure 8

Step 1: Stand in Starting Position.

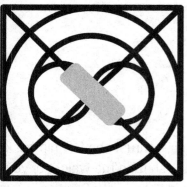

Step 2: Align the pelvis into Position 2.

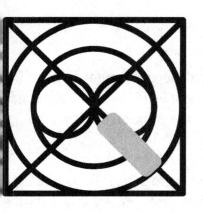

Step 3: Keeping the pelvis on the Position 2 axis, thrust the right hip backwards to the lower right corner of the outer circle. You will feel like you're sticking your butt out. To get the hip out far enough, you'll need to bend the right knee slightly while you keep the left leg straight.

If you don't bend your knees, you won't be able to move the hip out wide enough. Your weight will largely be supported by the right leg with the pelvis in this position.

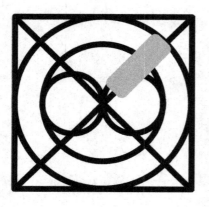

Step 4: Use the right hip to trace along the edge of the outer circle, moving the hip forward to the upper right corner of the map so that your pelvis is now aligned with Position 1. This motion should be exaggerated, almost like you are making a "scooping" motion. (It always reminds me of scooping out an avocado). Your pelvis is now in Position 1, with your right hip extended forward and your weight is largely supported on the right leg.

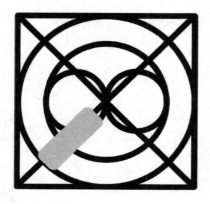

Step 5: Now reverse it. From Position 1, thrust the left hip backwards, bending the right knee slightly, shifting the weight of your body to the left leg, keeping the pelvis in line with Position 1.

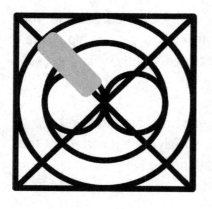

Step 6: "Scoop" the left hip forward along the outer circle to the upper left corner. Your pelvis will now be in Position 2 again and when you come back to center you've completed tracing the figure eight.

Step 7: Repeat the motion by returning to Step 3. Thrust the right hip backwards and continue Steps 3 to 7 repeatedly until the motion feels comfortable.

Backward Figure 8

This motion is the same as the above, just moving in the opposite direction.

Step 1: Stand in Starting Position.

Step 2: Align the pelvis into Position 1.

Step 3: Keeping the pelvis on the Position 1 axis, thrust the right hip forwards to the upper right corner of the outer circle. It will feel funny. The weight of your body will largely be supported by your right leg. To get the hip out far enough, you'll need to bend the right knee slightly while you keep the left leg straight. If you don't bend your knees, you won't be able to move the hip out far enough.

Step 4: Use the right hip to trace along the outer circle, scooping the hip backwards towards the lower right corner of the map, so that your pelvis is now aligned with Position 2.

Step 5: From Position 2, thrust the left hip forwards along the axis, bending the left knee slightly, pushing into the floor as you straighten the right leg, shifting the weight of the body to the left leg, keeping the pelvis in line with Position 2.

Step 6: "Scoop" the left hip backwards along the outer circle to the lower left corner. Your pelvis will now be in Position 1 again and when you come back to center you've completed tracing the figure 8.

Step 7: Repeat the motion by beginning with Step 3, thrust the right hip upwards to the right and repeat the steps again.

Level 3: Adding the Knees to the Figure 8

In Level 2, you started to see how the movement of the hips was enabled by the bending of the knees. In fact, the movement of the hips is entirely dependent upon the knees. If you don't bend the legs at the knee, it's impossible to move the hips beyond a slight shift of the pelvis. You can move the pelvis in a figure 8 motion inside the small inner circle, but to move it along the outside, you'll need to bend the knees.

Level 3 brings a higher level of attention to how the knees move.

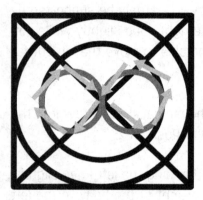

Step 1: Try to move your knees in a Forward Figure 8 by tracing the figure eight at the center of the Movement Map.

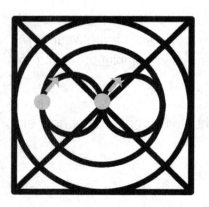

Most likely, you'll notice that you instinctively want to move your knees in parallel.

That's a good motion to practice, but that's not what we want here. We want the knees to move in opposition to each other, not in parallel.

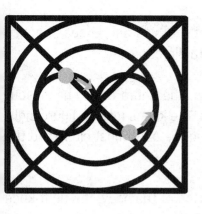

When the left knee is at the front of the left circle (or left half of the Figure 8), then the right knee is at the back of the right circle (or right half of the Figure 8), etc.

When your knees are in this position, notice that the right leg is straight and the left knee is bent, and the pelvis is in Position 2. When you move the knees around the circles to the other sides, the right knee is bent at the front, the left leg is straight with the knee at the back, and the pelvis is in Position 1. Discover how the position of the knees impacts the position of the hips.

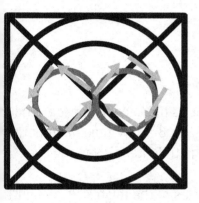

Step 2: Repeat the circular motion of the knees until it becomes comfortable.

Step 3: Continuing the motion, bring your attention to your hips. Notice how as the knee moves in a circle (either direction) the corresponding hip moves in a circle as well. Notice how the hip and knee are connected and move together as one. Keep repeating the figure eight motion and discover that you can move your knees by bringing your attention to your hips, and you can move your hips by bringing your attention to your knees. They are connected.

Step 4: Bend the knees slightly and notice how this exaggerates the motion of the knees and hips. It should make it easier to see how they are connected.

Step 5: Go back to Level 3 Step 1, and do a Backward Figure 8 with the knees. Continue to explore how the knees and hips are connected.

Step 8: Bend the knees a little more to exaggerate the motion of the hips and knees. Practice tracing a figure eight with the knees in both forward and backward directions.

With practice, you will discover that as you use your hips to trace the figure eight shape, your knees are making alternating circles to make a figure eight as well. The knees make a figure eight along the two inner-most circles; the hips make a figure eight using the outermost circle and the X axes.

When doing a Forward Figure 8, the knees circle towards the midline of the body: the right knee is moving counterclockwise and the left clockwise. When doing a Backwards Figure 8, the knees circle away from the midline of the body: the right knee moves clockwise and the left counter-clockwise.

Putting it all Together

Now that you've mastered the motion of the lower body, notice that as the knee of one leg bends, the knee of the opposite leg straightens. Perform the Forward Figure 8 a few times and notice how one leg straightens as the other bends, and then the other leg straightens, over and over.

As each leg straightens, push down into the floor. Engage the muscles of the thigh, calf, and butt. Push down into the floor to propel the scooping and thrusting of the pelvis. With the pelvis in Position 1, you can trace a straight line from the heel of the left foot up the straightened leg and out the right hip in Position 1. Feel the movement of the toes, the ankle joint, the knees and the hips. Squeeze the muscles of the butt as you thrust the hip. Squeeze the knee caps as the legs bend and straighten. Tighten the abdominals to energize the core. Place your hands on your hips and notice the motion of the elbows. Bring your consciousness to every part of your body as you move. Practice the movement both forward and backward.

Over time, your intellect will be required less and your body will create the motion effortlessly and automatically. The pleasure of this miraculous movement will become your gift to yourself, every single morning for the rest of your life.

MOVEMENT INFORMATION

Movement Name
Figure 8

Difficulty
Level 1 (The Twist)
Level 2 (Moving the Hips in a Figure 8)
Level 3 (The complete movement with hips and knees together)

Where you'll see it
Latin and Cuban dance: Samba, Merengue, Salsa, etc.
Belly Dancing: "horizontal figure eight hip roll."

What it wakes up
Everything from the chest down.

Contraindications and Cautions
If performed carelessly, this motion can put excess pressure on the spine and lower back.
Move from the pelvis, keeping the core stable; don't twist from the spine.

Deepen the Movement
Bend the knees while performing this movement, so as to drop down into a Figure 8 dynamic squat. This motion works in both forward and backward movements. When performing this motion, do not go lower than you feel confident.

In the Beginning...
Don't overthink it. Just have fun and practice daily. Get an instructor or friend to help. This

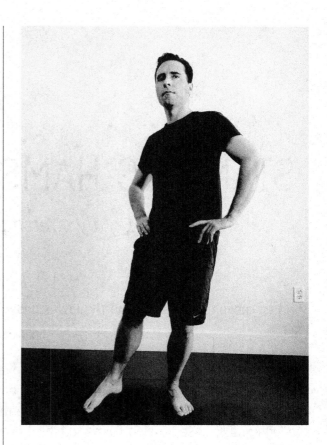

motion is easier to learn in person.

Additional Research
Search: "How to do Cuban Motion"
Search: "How to do Belly Dancing Horizontal Figure Eight with Hips"
Search: "Belly Dancing Twist" and other Belly Dancing tutorials.

2.

STANDING HAMSTRING STRETCH

Lightly stretch the hamstrings.

The last movement warmed up the lower body. This motion will lightly stretch the backs of the legs.

The Standing Hamstring Stretch is a simple movement where the heel is extended in front of the body and the opposite leg is bent to pull the hamstring of the extended leg. It's held for only a second before switching to the other leg. The motion is repeated several times to fully awaken the legs and release tension from the hips. I find this motion releases tension in the lower back as well, warming up my back for any bending that my day requires.

Step By Step

Step 1: Extend your right leg and place the back of the right heel on the floor in front of you. Point your toes up to the ceiling, or even better, up and back towards your forehead.

Step 2: Drop your butt down towards the floor, bending the left knee slightly, keeping your right heel firmly planted in the floor and your right leg straight.

Step 3: Feel the stretch through the entire right hamstring. Most often the stretch will be felt in the calf or right behind the knee. To deepen the stretch where it matters, arch the back slightly so you stick out your butt. This will allow you to feel the stretch at the top of the leg where it meets the pelvis, reducing a lot of tension where you didn't even know you had it.

Caution: Be sure not to overstretch or hold the pose for too long.

Step 4: Come back up to standing position and repeat the same steps using the opposite leg.

Step 5: Once you get the hang of the motion, alternate from one leg to the other in a smooth motion, holding the stretch for just a second or two before moving to the opposite leg. This will ensure you don't over-stretch, and it makes this a dynamic and pleasurable movement instead of a painful static stretch.

MOVEMENT INFORMATION

Movement Name
Standing Hamstring Stretch

Difficulty
Level 1

Where you'll see it
Stretching
Physical Therapy
What it wakes up
Hamstrings
Knees
Feet

Contraindications and Cautions
Do not stretch to the point of discomfort
or pain.

Deepen the Movement
Bend the knee deeply in order to approach or
achieve a one-legged squat.

In the Beginning...
Use a chair to keep your balance if you are
concerned about falling.

Additional Research
Search: "Standing Hamstring Stretch"
Search: "Cossack Squat" or "Archer Squat"

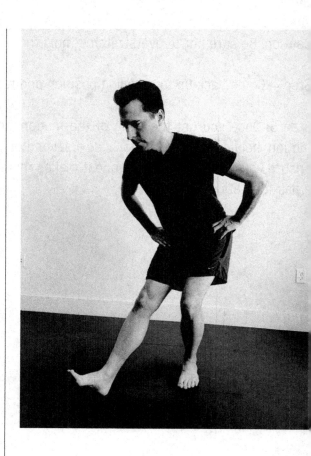

3. TORSO TWISTS

Twist your upper torso from side to side while keeping the pelvis stable and forward-facing.

At this point in the sequence, you've awakened the legs and the core. It's now time to engage the arms and upper torso, including the upper spine and back. The Torso Twist is a gentle but powerful way to energize the spine and wakeup the arms and chest. This motion stimulates the circulatory and digestive systems, strengthens the abdomen, and increases range of motion in the spine. It also wakes up the joints of the arms, including the wrists, elbows, and fingers.

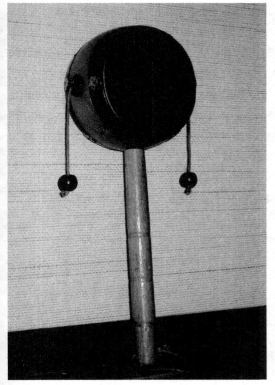

You've probably seen a traditional exercise called a Torso Twist where a broom is placed on the shoulders, the arms are wrapped around, and the torso is twisted from side to side. This movement terrifies me and you should never do it unless under the supervision of a doctor. It puts way too much pressure on the lower back, and it tends to be executed in a careless manner, further risking injury.

In our version of the Torso Twist, we only twist the upper torso, keeping the lower back stable and stationary. The pelvis faces forward through the whole movement, and only the chest moves from side to side.

When first learning the movement, sit on a chair and rotate the upper body from side to side. Your hips won't be able to move, so you'll learn how the movement feels.

As you advance, drop the arms to the sides and let them flop around like a rag doll. Discover how the chest can propel the arms to move from side to side around the chest and back.

The easiest way to visualize this motion is to picture a child's toy pellet drum. A pellet drum is a percussion instrument, comprised of a two-sided drum on a stick. On either side of the drum are two pellets attached with string. When the drum is twisted from side to side, the motion propels the pellets outward and they beat the drum. This is the motion you want to imitate. Rotate the torso powerfully so that the arms are propelled to beat on your chest and back.

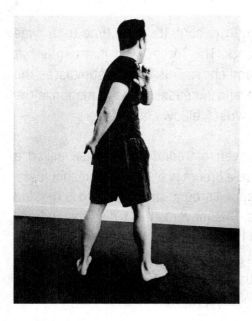

Step By Step

Step 1: Begin in Starting Position with the hands on the hips.

Step 2: Move the torso back and forth repeatedly from Position 1 to Position 2 to loosen the upper spine and chest.

Step 3: Drop the arms to the sides and let them hang loose like a rag doll. Thrust the upper torso from Position 2 to Position 1, and feel how when you do this the left arm swings to the right side of the body, and the right arm swings behind you. Repeat the motion the opposite direction, and observe the motion of the arms.

Step 4: Intensify the motion of the torso, propelling the arms in front of and behind you.

Step 5: Repeat this motion several times until your upper body feels loose and awake.

MOVEMENT INFORMATION

Movement Name
Torso Twist

Difficulty
Level 2

Where you'll see it
An abdominal exercise called "Russian Twist"
Torso rotations
Torso rotation machines

What it wakes up
Lower and upper back muscles
Spine and neck
Elbows, hands and wrists
Abdominals

Contraindications and Cautions
If not performed carefully this can be a dangerous movement, causing damage to the lower back/spine. Move slowly and intentionally at all times, supporting the lower back with the abdominals, and keeping the pelvis stable so as to prevent over-extension of the spine.
If you have any type of back pain or injury, do not perform this movement without the supervision and permission of a doctor.
Move slowly. At no time should you feel any pain or discomfort.
If you have any concerns about your back, adjust the movement so that you move the arms from side to side.

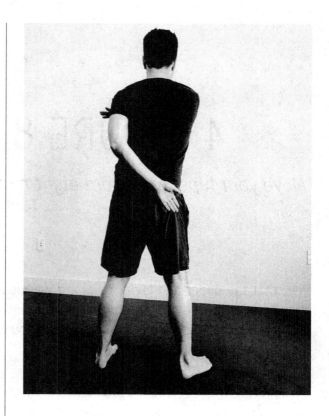

Deepen the Movement
None needed.
In the Beginning…
Be gentle. Discover how the arm movement is an extension of the twisting of the torso. Don't overdo it.

Additional Research
Search: "Russian Twist Exercise"
Search: "Standing Oblique Twist" (This is what you do not want to do; it places too much pressure on the spine).

4. FIGURE 8 WITH ARMS

Move your hips in a figure eight motion, propelling the arms from side to side.

Now that the upper and lower body are warmed-up, it's time to bring everything you've learned already (yes, it's been a lot) together in one motion. In Movement 1, you learned to move the hips in a figure eight motion, and in Movement 3, you learned to move the torso back and forth to beat the arms against the chest and back.

The Figure 8 with Arms is a combination of Movements 1 and 3.

Move the hips in Forward Figure 8, and let the motion of the hips propel the twisting of the torso and the movement of the arms.

When done properly, this movement is elegant, energizing, and liberating. There is a Hindu concept called "Kundalini," which is described as an energizing force located at the base of the spine. Often described as a snake, when the Kundalini is awakened, the body feels ecstatic rushes of energy throughout it.

Step By Step

Step 1: Start out doing a Forward Figure 8.

Step 2: Let the arms hang loose at the sides like a rag-doll.

Allow yourself to feel the motion of your hips and pelvis throughout your body, particularly your torso.

Step 3: Gently allow your hands to "flop" loosely from side to side as your hips move. This motion will mimic the arm motions of the Torso Twist, only you'll just be doing them low and loose. Discover how the flapping motion originates in the figure eight movement of the pelvis.

Step 4: As you fully understand how the movement of the pelvis causes your arms to move, intensify the arm movement, slapping them higher and higher on the body, all the time as a result of the motion of the pelvis.

Step 5: As you fully engage, you will be simultaneously doing the Forward Figure 8 on your lower body, while your arms and upper torso will be doing a Torso Twist.

MOVEMENT INFORMATION

Movement Name
Figure 8 with Arms

Difficulty
Level 3

Where you'll see it
To my knowledge, only TheraQi. If you have seen this movement elsewhere, please tell me about it.

What it wakes up
Everything

Contraindications and Cautions
If not performed carefully this can be a dangerous movement, causing damage to the lower back/spine. Move slowly and intentionally at all times, supporting the lower back with the abdominals, and keeping the pelvis stable so as to prevent over-extension of the spine. If you have any type of back pain or injury, do not perform this movement without the supervision and permission of a doctor. Move slowly. At no time should you feel any pain or discomfort.
If you have any concerns about your back, adjust the movement so that you move the arms from side to side.

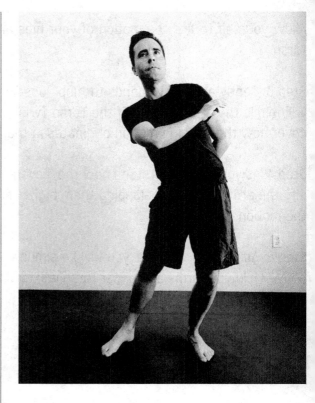

Deepen the Movement
Increase the intensity of the motion and push down deeply into the ground to propel the body.
Experiment with variations of your own.

In the Beginning...
Do not get frustrated if the move doesn't come easily. It's one of the most complex movements in the sequence.

Additional Research
This is a move best studied in person with an instructor or another person who has mastered the movement.

5. HEAD HULA

Slide your head in a circle without turning or tilting.

The entire body is lightly awakened, the spine is loose, and it's time to go deeper into awakening specific parts of the body through isolations. In Head Hula, we discover more about how to awaken the head and neck for releasing tension, increasing range of motion, and preventing injury.

Using soup cans, let's take a closer look at three ways the head can move. The first two are obvious, but the third will probably new. For the sake of this exercise, visualize the vertebrae in your spine as two soup cans stacked on top of each other.

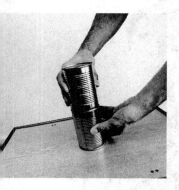

First, the soup cans can turn (or twist) from side to side. (Notice the seams of the cans are pointing in different directions). We turn the head every time we look over our shoulder, or when we check our blind spot while driving.

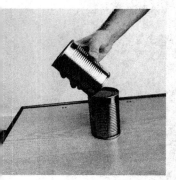

Second, the soup cans can tilt from side to side, as if the top can is being poured out. The head can also tilt, and by tiling in all directions, can make a circle. This "head circle" motion is called a neck roll, and is a standard movement in yoga and other warmup programs.

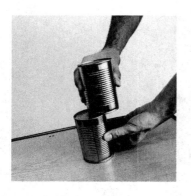

The third way the cans can move is in a slide. In a slide, the top can stays flat against the bottom; the front of the can stays facing forward; and the can moves in a circle around the circumference of the lower can.

The head can make a similar motion, sliding in a circle while pointing straight ahead, and keeping the midline of the head perpendicular to the floor. The chest and pelvis can make this sliding motion as well. The easiest way I've found to communicate this complex circular-sliding motion is by associating it with the Hula. Hula dancing and Hula hooping both rely heavily on these types of slides, and since Hula is a familiar concept to the average person, it seems like the easiest way to explain a complex idea.

Hula hooping is a wonderful form of exercise, and it's unfortunate that it's no longer as popular as it used to be. Hula creates a rotational force sufficient to keep the hoop aloft by pulsing the pelvis (or chest or head) in a very small circle. Hula is not a twist; the body remains positioned forward at all times. Hula is also not a tilt; if the body tilts the hoop will fall off.

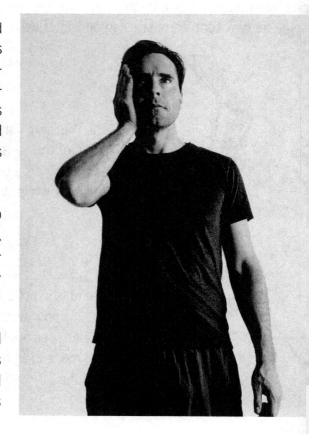

The easiest way to learn how to Head Hula is to place your hand against the side of your head, and press your face against your hand. The muscles you use to press are the same ones to engage with the hand down.

Learning to isolate the pelvis, chest, and head and move them Hula-style opens up your body's self-expression and leaves you with style and grace when you move. As an athlete, it unlocks your spine and prevents injury. And for all of us, Hula just feels good. It energizes the spine and leaves you feeling awake and relaxed. Head Hula reduces pain in the neck and shoulders, reduces tension in the scalp, and reduces the risk of injury while performing daily tasks.

The only thing to be careful of in any type of Hula is doing too many Hulas at a time, or doing them too deeply before the range of motion has widened. Don't push yourself. Be gentle and enjoy.

Step By Step

Step 1: Look in the mirror and practice the following endpoints of a Head Hula circle:

Place your hand on your forehead, and press the forehead against the hand. Remove the hand and repeat the press, this time jutting the head forward then pulling it back.

Place your hand on the right side of your head and press into it. Remove the hand and slide your head to the right, keeping the face forward and the midline of the head perpendicular to the ground. (Don't tilt).

Slide the head back, making sure you face forward, don't lift the chin.

Place the left hand against the left side of the head, and press into it. Remove the hand and slide the head to the left, keeping the face pointed forward and the midline of the head perpendicular to the ground.

Step 2: Once you have a sense of your forward/back/left/right endpoints, and you're comfortable extending to those points, connect them in a circle: front, right, back, left, front. Repeat this motion a couple of times, being careful to not overextend.

Step 3: Reverse the direction of the circle and repeat. Over time, the motion will become smooth and easy.

MOVEMENT INFORMATION

Movement Name
Head Hula

Difficulty
Level 3

Where you'll see it
Belly dancing
Break dancing
Hula hooping
What it wakes up
Head
Neck

Contraindications and Cautions
If not performed carefully this can be a dangerous movement, causing damage to the neck and spine. Move slowly and intentionally at all times, keeping the head stable.
If you have any type of neck pain or injury, do not perform this movement without the supervision and permission of a doctor.
Move slowly. At no time should you feel any pain or discomfort.
Do not over-extend. Small is better.

Deepen the Movement
Do not deepen this movement, you may risk injury. Focus on perfecting the form and smoothness of the movement.

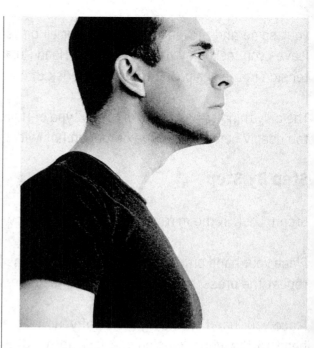

In the Beginning...
Hold a cup under your chin and trace the rim of the cup to guide the movement of the head.

Additional Research
Search: "Belly Dancing Neck Slide" or "Belly Dancing Head Slide"

6.
SHOULDER CIRCLES

Make circles with the shoulders.

Working our way down the body we next arrive at the shoulders.

The shoulders are magical things. They move in so many directions and take more abuse from our body than they deserve. At the same time, they are extremely fragile. Shoulder pain and locked shoulders are a common complaint. Shoulder Circles are a simple exercise, but for those plagued with shoulder injuries this exercise can be difficult to achieve.

To complete this movement, make circles backwards with both shoulders simultaneously, then forwards simultaneously, then alternating backwards, then alternating forwards.

Shoulder Circles release the tension in the upper back, chest, and clavicle areas, and will leave you feeling like you've just gotten a massage.

Step By Step

Step 1: Move the shoulders together, simultaneously in a backward circle. Repeat the motion several times, deepening it as you go.

Step 2: Then switch directions and move the shoulders in a forward motion. Repeat the motion several times.

Step 3: Move the shoulders in alternating circles moving backward, one shoulder at a time. (When one shoulder is moving, the other is still).

Step 4: Move the shoulders in alternating circles moving forward, one shoulder at a time. (When one shoulder is moving, the other is still).

Step 5: Move the shoulders in alternating circles moving backward, but this time have both shoulders move simultaneously, as if you are trying to swim in the water with only your shoulders. Notice how the shoulders move opposite each other. When one shoulder is up the other is down, and when one is forward the other is backwards. Repeat the motion several times.

Step 6: Move the shoulders in alternating (but simultaneous) circles moving forward. Again, notice how the shoulders are opposite each other. Repeat the motion several times before moving to the next movement.

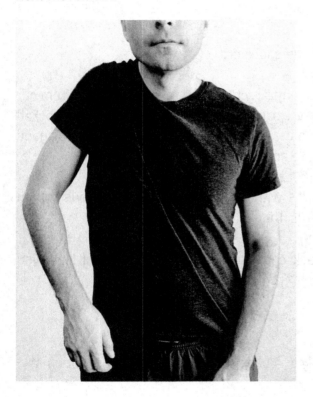

MOVEMENT INFORMATION

Movement Name
Shoulder Circles

Difficulty
Level 1

Where you'll see it
Typical warmup exercises
Shoulder shrugs in weightlifting

What it wakes up
Shoulders
Chest
Upper back

Contraindications and Cautions
This is a generally safe movement.
Go slow and end the movement if you en-
counter any pain.
If you have any popping of the shoulder,
adjust the movement to avoid popping.

Deepen the Movement
Add weight to intensify the movement.

In the Beginning...
Use a mirror to check your form.

Additional Research
Search: "Shoulder shrugs" or "Shoulder circles"

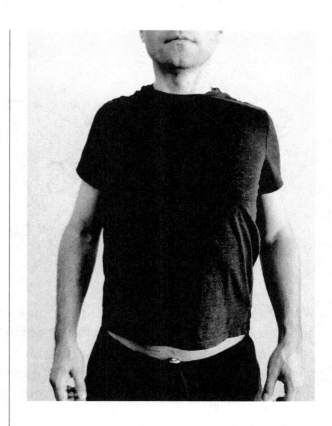

7.
PUSHES AND PULLS

Push your arms out and pull them back in.

With the shoulder joints loosened up, we next move to awaken the expanded clavicle area: not only the shoulder joint, but also the muscles of the shoulders, chest, and upper back. Nearly every upper body activity depends on these muscles and the movement of these joints. The upper body and how it moves up, out, down and around is essential to the successful performance of our daily routines: carrying groceries, reaching up to get something off a shelf, starting a lawn mower, etc.

We need our shoulder area to be strong and flexible. The traditional way of building upper body strength is by going to a gym and lifting weights. But many people, myself included, struggle to feel comfortable in a gym. There are so many machines… and what exactly are you supposed to do with all those dumbbells?

This chapter aims to explain upper body strength training using the TheraQi method. By the end of the chapter you will learn 10 key upper body exercises, and never feel too intimidated to visit a gym again. And, if like me, you choose not to lift weights, you will get a powerful and energizing new way to stretch and tone your upper body.

Pushing and Pulling: The Keys to Strength

All weight training can be distilled down to two simple tasks: push heavy things away from your body and pull heavy things towards your body. The fancy terms for these movements are "extending" and "flexing." When weight is pushed away from the body, it's extending. When weight is lled towards the body, it's flexing.

r example, a bench press and an overhead dumbbell press are two ways of pushing weight
vay from the body. Pushing can also happen when you push your body away from a stationary
ject, such as the floor, like in a push-up. Another example is a dip, where you push against bars,
gs, handles, or other stationary objects to raise and lower your body.

amples of pulling weight towards the body include a deadlift, a bicep curl, and a cable pull.
amples of when you pull your body towards a stationary object include exercising on a rowing
ichine and doing pull-ups.

interesting that when you push or pull the movement of the body is basically the same. When
u do a push up and when you row on a rowing machine, you are essentially executing the same
vement. In one instance you're pulling and in the other you're pushing.

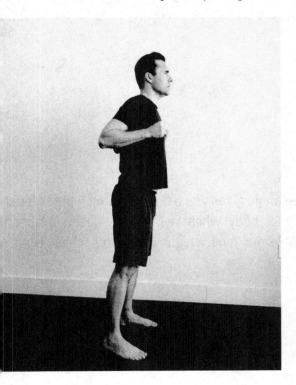

For example, in this picture, have I just finished rowing or am I about to do a push-up?

The movements are the same, but the muscle groups used to push versus pull are different.

It's the same with a pull-up and an overhead dumbbell press—same movement, different muscles. Almost any time you do a push exercise, there's a corresponding pull to go with it and vice versa. By combining push and pull exercises, you can create a balanced weightlifting routine.

Pushing and Pulling in the Gym:
The Five Angles of Upper Body Fitness

Once you understand the principles of pushing and pulling, the gym stops being such a scary place. Just change the angle of your arms to your body, and you unlock a range of different exercises. There are five key angles to know about. I call these different arm angles "The Five Angles of Uppder Body Fitness" because they provide the foundation for a majority of upper body exercises you will see in a gym or that you would do with a trainer.

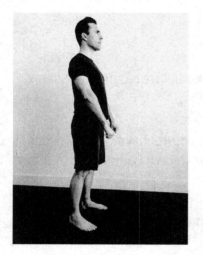

Here are each of the Five Angles of Upper Body Fitness and what strength training exercises they enable:

Angle #1: A zero degree angle, with the arms down at your sides or right in front of the hips, gives you a dip (push yourself up from a stationary object) and a chin-raise (pull weight up to your chin).

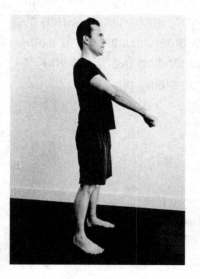

Angle #2: A 45 degree angle gives you a declined bench press (push weight away from your body while laying on a declined bench) and a lower-level cable pull (pull weight up to your chest from a floor-level cable).

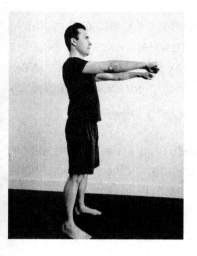

Angle #3: A 90 degree angle gives you a push-up (push your body away from the floor) or bench press (push weight away from the chest) and a row (pull weight towards your body, or pull your body forward like on a rowing machine).

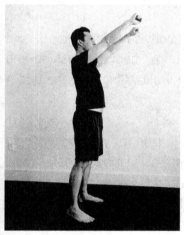

Angle #4: A 135 degree angle gives you an inclined bench press (push) and an overhead cable pull (pull).

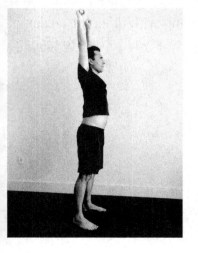

Angle #5: A 180 degree angle (arms overhead) gives you an overhead press (push weight up overhead) and a pull-up (pull yourself up via a stationary object such as a bar or rope).

When you push and pull at each of the five angles, you end up with ten exercises (five angles multiplied by two directions of force, equals ten total movements).

These ten exercises are the only upper body weightlifting exercises you will ever need to know. These simple moves will give you a lifetime of exercise. Experiment with different ways of pushing and pulling at those angles and you will have unlimited methods to stay strong. You can even experiment with finding ways to do them around the house (such as working purely with your body weight or pushing and pulling common objects).

Pushing and pulling are the only two ways of building muscle and strength. These two simple activities are the primary ways our bodies express their power, and understanding how your body moves when you push and pull will expand your ability to build muscle and burn fat.

Pushing and Pulling in TheraQi

Before you ever push or pull heavy weight, you need to wake up your body's muscles, joints, and other biological systems. In the TheraQi sequence, we wake up the upper body by pushing and pulling our arms into the air at each of the five angles. And to really wake things up, we add a rotation to the arms while we push and pull.

Stop reading for a moment and do this little test: push your arm out in front of your body (Angle #3) and stick out your thumb. Which way is your thumb pointing? If you're like most people, it will naturally be pointing to the midline of the body, or inward and downward towards the floor. With your arm still out, rotate your arm so that your thumb traces the full range of motion: inward all the way, pointing down perpendicular to the floor; inward parallel to the floor; upward towards the ceiling; and outward parallel to the floor. Are any of these positions easier or harder for you? Moving your arms in a pushing and pulling motion while experimenting with different angles of rotation is an excellent way to expand your range of motion and improve your ability to manage heavy weight.

Learning to Rotate: Step by Step

Step 1: Extend your arms out in front of you in the Angle #3 (90 degrees), make a fist, and stick out your thumbs towards the ceiling. You can also grab a pencil or a kitchen utensil to help you visualize the rotation.

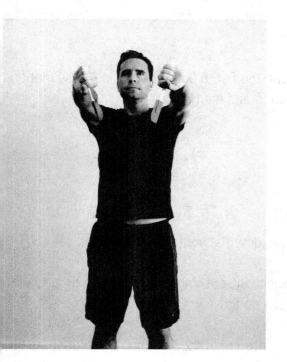
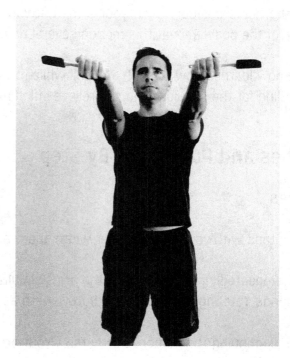

Step 2: Now turn the fists in towards the midline of the body and downward to the floor.

Step 3: Then rotate the thumbs up and outward.

Step 4: Repeat this motion a few times—inward, then rotate outward, then back.

Step 5: Now pull the fists in towards the body, raising the thumb/pencil/spatula as you pull back. By the time the fists reach your shoulders, the thumb will be pointing up. This is the "home position" for all pushing and pulling movements, regardless of which of the Five Angles of Upper Body Fitness you are moving in.

Step 6: Practice moving from the home position to Angle #3 several times, rotating your fists downward and inward as you push. You'll be pointing inward/downward when you have the arms extended, and upward when you come back to home. Repeat this motion several times.

Step 7: Keep pushing outward and returning to home, but switch the direction of the rotation. From the home position, push your arms outwards, rotating the fists outward away from the midline of the body. Repeat this motion several times.

You've now learned how to push and pull while rotating the fist in both directions. These motions are healing for the shoulder and can relieve inflammation and injury.

Pushes and Pulls: Step By Step

Pushes

Step 1: Stand with your feet shoulder width apart, arms down at your sides (Angle #1).

Step 2: Repeatedly raise and lower the arms simultaneously, pushing down into the ground with both hands, rotating the fists inward/downward as you do so.

Step 3: Continuing the motion, slowly raise your arms into Angle #2. Continue the motion at this angle a few times.

Step 4: Repeat the above at Angle #3; then #4, then #5 until you are pushing/punching with your arms overhead.

Step 5: After repeating the motion a few times, begin to lower the arms, continuing the punching motion through Angle #4, #3, #2 and back to #1.

Step 6: Repeat the steps above, rotating the fists outward this time.

Alternating Pushes

Step 7: Repeat Steps 1 to 6 above, only this time, alternate the arms. Lock the elbows tightly on the extension. Be sure to move the rotation in both directions.

Pulls

Step 8: Go back to home position. Repeat Steps 1 through 6 above, this time focusing on the pulling motion. Pretend you are rowing or pulling on a rope. You'll feel different muscles being used, and your hands may instinctively reach or grab for imaginary handles. Repeat these motions a few times until your upper body is awake.

MOVEMENT INFORMATION

Movement Name
Pushes and Pulls

Difficulty
Level 2

Where you'll see it
Wide-grip pull-ups in weightlifting
Boxing/martial arts
Shoulder press with dumbbells
Lat pull-downs
Pushups

What it wakes up
Upper and lower back
Chest
Arms, shoulders, elbows and wrists
Abdominals

Contraindications and Cautions
This is a generally safe movement. Go slow and end the movement if you encounter any pain. If you have any popping of the shoulder, adjust the movement to avoid popping.

Deepen the Movement
Alternate arms to study the different ways your body moves.

Increase the intensity of the movement to make more of an aerobic exercise and increase the heart rate.

When you're ready, go to the gym once or twice a week and experiment with adding weight to further study this movement. Add-

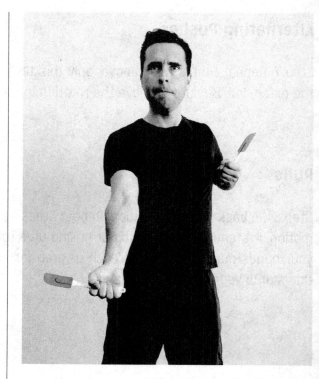

ing weight to a movement has two key benefits: first, it allows you to benefit from the additional exertion required. Second, the weight serves as a diagnostic to help you "stress test" your form. The movement will become easier when you put the weight down.

In the Beginning...
Place a pencil or some other object in your curled up fists to make the twisting of the wrist more visible.

Additional Research
Watch videos on various upper body free weight exercises to better understand the motions discussed.

8.
BUTTERFLY PRESS

Move your arms forward and back with elbows at right angles.

In the previous movement, you learned how to move the arms at different angles. This movement builds on that idea. The Butterfly Press is a movement performed at multiple angles along the torso. You start with the arms to the sides and slowly raise them up along the side of the body (not the front) until they are overhead.

The Butterfly Press and its opposite, the Reverse Butterfly, are good movements to open the shoulders, shoulder girdle, and upper back.

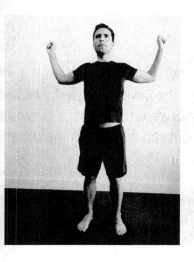 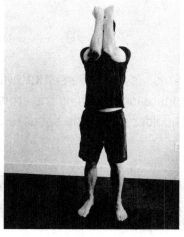

Butterfly Press

The Butterfly Press begins with the lower arms raised to the sides, with the upper arms pointing up towards the ceiling.

To complete the press, bring the upper arms together in front of the midline of the body.

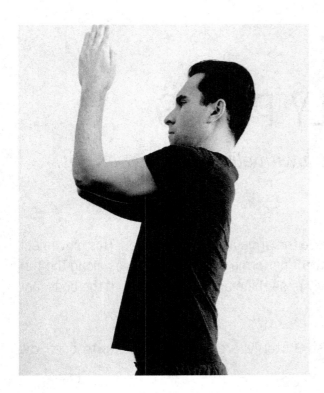

The challenge of the Butterfly Press is in trying to keep the arms at 90 degree angles when they are pressed together. Notice how when you bring the arms together in the press, your elbows may want to spread open, your upper arms will point down to the floor, and your hands will point towards your face.

The value of the Butterfly Press is in resisting these natural tendencies to collapse the arms. Instead, work to squeeze the elbows together, raise the elbows/upper arms parallel to the floor, and point the hands up to the ceiling rather than the face.

Doing so will open up the upper back and stretch out the shoulders.

Reverse Butterfly

The opposite movement of a Butterfly Press is the Reverse Butterfly. The Reverse Butterfly has a similar form to the Butterfly Press, but instead of pushing the arms forward towards the midline, pull them behind you to open up the shoulder girdle and squeeze tight the muscles in the upper back.

I love this movement because it moves the shoulders in ways we don't normally expect. It's relatively normal to think of moving the shoulders up down (like a shrug). In this movement we push the shoulders forwards and backwards. If you've done the Shoulder Circles earlier in the sequence, then this movement should come easily to you.

Step By Step

Step 1: Stand with feet shoulder width apart, arms extended down to the sides, hands rolled into fists.

Step 2: Thrust the shoulders and arms backwards, as though you're trying to squeeze a credit card between your shoulder blades.

Step 3: Relax and repeat several times.

Step 4: Keep repeating the motion, and as you do so, raise the arms up to your sides, slowly, until your arms are in the Butterfly Press Starting Position. Keep repeating the Reverse Butterfly as you raise the arms, so that you perform the motion at several angles along the way to the Butterfly Press position.

Step 5: When you reach 90 degrees, switch directions and do a Butterfly Press. Bring the arms together, squeezing the elbows together, trying your best to keep the arms raised up and outward towards the ceiling.

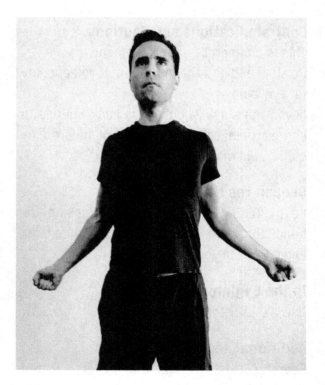

Step 6: Open the arms and repeat the Butterfly Press a few times.

Step 7: Go back to doing the Reverse Butterfly, and continue raising the arms until they are overhead. The further up your arms go, the more awkward the movement will feel, but just keep doing your best to thrust the shoulders and arms behind you. Stop when you get the arms fully overhead.

MOVEMENT INFORMATION

Movement Name
Butterfly Press

Difficulty
Level 1

Where you'll see it
Weightlifting/Bodybuilding
Eagle Pose in yoga
What it wakes up
Back
Chest
Arms, elbows, shoulders

Contraindications and Cautions
This is a generally safe movement.
Go slow and end the movement if you encounter any pain.
If you have any shoulder or back injuries or chronic pain, talk to your doctor before executing this movement.

Deepen the Movement
Keep 90 degree angles when pressing the hands together. If you master it, go on to learn Eagle Pose in yoga.

In the Beginning...
Use a mirror to check your form.

Additional Research
Search: "Butterfly Press" and "Reverse Butterfly Press"
Search: "Eagle Pose Yoga"

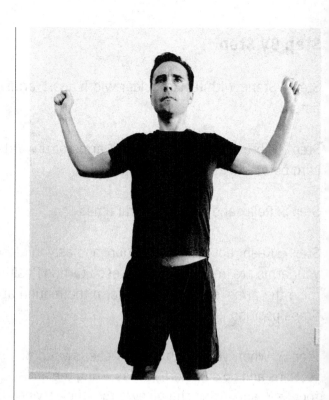

9. OVERHEAD STRETCH

Reach your arms overhead, fingers interlaced, and stretch.

We ended the Butterfly Press with the arms up overhead. Once they are there, it's time to stretch them deeply.

The Overhead Stretch is a simple, effective exercise for stimulating the arms and torso.

I love how the Overhead Stretch releases tension in the ribcage and arms while strengthening the shoulders. It also releases tension in the hands and wrists, and improves overall posture by elongating the torso.

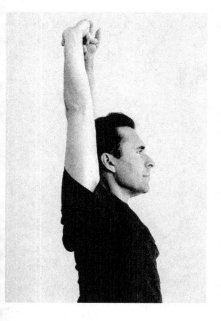

Step By Step

Step 1: Stand in Starting Position.

Step 2: Raise your arms overhead; interlace the fingers with palms facing up towards the ceiling and tighten the elbows. Stretch the fingers and press the shoulders down to deepen the stretch in the arms.

Step 3: Bring the hands down far enough to switch the position of the fingers. If the left index finger was on top, put the right index finger on top instead. Repeat Step 2 above using the new finger placement.

Step 4: Hold for a few counts and then lower your arms enough to flip the hands around so the fingers are interlaced with the palms together, then stretch overhead again.

Step 4: Gently move your arms from side to side, left to right. You'll feel the stretch through the sides of your ribcage.

Step 5: Repeat a couple of times with both hand positions and then relax.

MOVEMENT INFORMATION

Movement Name
Overhead Stretch

Difficulty
Level 1

Where you'll see it
Warmup
Steeple Stretch and/or Tree Pose in Yoga
What it wakes up
Hands, wrists, fingers
Biceps, triceps, shoulders
Back muscles

Contraindications and Cautions
This is a generally safe movement.
Go slow and end the movement if you encounter any pain.
If you have any shoulder or back injuries or chronic pain, talk to your doctor before executing this movement.

Deepen the Movement
The intensity of this movement comes from the degree to which you push the shoulders down and reach the arms up.
You can also intensify it by holding the pose for longer periods of time.

In the Beginning...
Use a mirror to check your form.
If you struggle with this movement, lay down on your back and reach up overhead while lying down. It's the same movement just a dif-

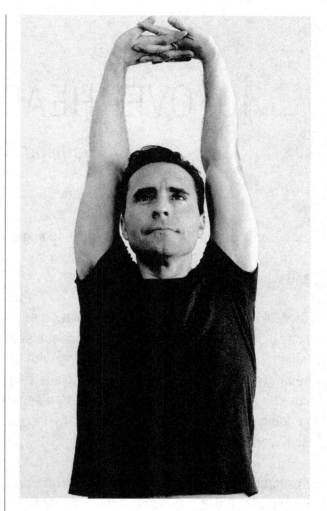

ferent position. The floor will serve as a clear line of whether or not you are able to reach overhead.

Additional Research
Search: "Steeple Stretch for Back Pain"

10. OVERHEAD CHEST HULA

Stretch overhead and hula your chest.

Let's continue the overhead theme by adding a Chest Hula to the overhead stretch. You already learned one Hula movement, the Head Hula. This chapter expands on what the Hula is all about and why it matters.

TheraQi is built on a foundation of isolation movements. Isolations are when a specific part of the body is moved separately from movement elsewhere in the body. Advanced dancers can combine isolations in one dance, to do one thing with one part of the body while doing something totally separate with another part. For example, a belly dancer may isolate the pelvis (doing a Figure 8), but she might also isolate the hands in a separate movement. This ability to combine isolations in complex ways is a signature of many types of dance, such as ballet, jazz, belly dancing, and Bollywood-style dance.

In addition to waking up various muscle groups, isolation exercises help develop control of specific body parts. This is a good exercise not only for the body but for the brain. Isolations tend to greatly expand not only control of motion but also range of motion. This improves flexibility, coordination and one's overall ability to move freely and with grace. In short, isolations keep you young.

As enjoyable as they are, isolations can be tricky to learn, since most of us have spent our lives without doing them. Our bodies are literally locked up. The chest isolation, Movement 15 "Chest Hula," in particular can be a challenge for many people. To make learning the chest isolation easier, we first learn the Overhead Chest Hula, in which the arms are lifted overhead. The arms in this position exaggerate the circular hula motion and make it easier to isolate the chest.

The average person has trouble bringing the arms straight up overhead and holding them behind the ears. Many people's arms lean forward in front of the body. In order to maximize the movement, push the arms straight up towards the ceiling, with the biceps resting right behind the ears.

Step By Step

Step 1: Raise the arms overhead with the fingers clasped, palms together (Overhead Stretch).

Step 2: Keeping the hips stationary and the abdominals tight, trace an imaginary circle on the ceiling using the hands. Alternatively, if you have your Movement Map on the floor, trace the outer circle with the hands.

Step 3: Engage the shoulders to "lock" the arms and shoulders in a stable position. This will force you to move from the chest, rather than the shoulders. You will feel the chest opening and expanding in all directions. Do several circles in one direction, and then reverse directions for several more.

MOVEMENT INFORMATION

Movement Name
Chest Circles Plus Overhead Stretch

Difficulty
Level 2

Where you'll see it
Stretching
Hula hooping
Jazz dance
What it wakes up
Arms
Chest
Back

Contraindications and Cautions
If not performed carefully this can be a dangerous movement, causing damage to the spine. Move slowly and intentionally at all times, keeping the head stable.
If you have any type of back or neck pain or injury, do not perform this movement without the supervision and permission of a doctor.
Move slowly. At no time should you feel any pain or discomfort.
Do not over-extend. Small is better.

Deepen the Movement
Keep the elbows straightened and placed behind the ears. Do not lean forward.

In the Beginning...
Use a mirror to check your form.
Sit on the edge of a stiff flat chair when first

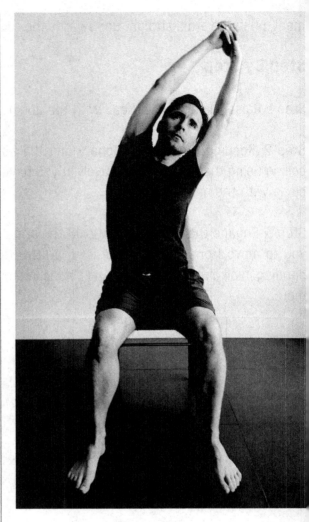

learning this movement. The chair will keep the hips from moving, allowing you to focus on the upper body.

Additional Research
Search: "How to Hula Hoop around the Chest"
Search: "Steeple Pose Yoga"

11. HIP HINGE AND HANG

Bend over with a straight back, and then hang upside down.

You've had your arms overhead for many movements now. You stretched them and then did several circles with the chest. Your arms are tired and you naturally want to bend over to relax from this overhead extension. In this chapter we discuss how to bend in a safe and comfortable manner to relax and prevent injury during everyday tasks.

The average person bends over countless times a day: picking up the laundry, the kids, the pets, weeding in the garden, picking up dirty clothes from the floor—it never ends. If you decide to weight-train, you have numerous bends in the gym, from toe touches to deadlifts. Most people bend in a totally unhealthy way, putting excess herniating strain on their spinal discs. This is the cause of back pain. It's preventable if you know how to bend.

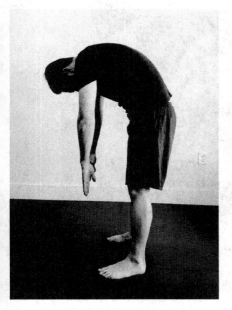

We often hear people say that the proper way to bend over is to "bend at the knees," but this is only part of the story. Not only do we need to bend the knees, we need to not bend the back. Wait, bending over without bending the back? It sounds impossible.

It is not!

The key is to "hinge" at the hip. Hinging means reducing the angle between the thigh and the lower abdomen.

Here's a photo of bending from the back without a hinge.

Notice how the angle between the thigh and the lower abdomen has not noticeably reduced; it's essentially still 180 degrees.

By bending the knees and hinging at the hips, the upper body can be lowered quite far without bending the spine. When the spine eventually does bend, it's "draped" across the tops of the thighs. The thighs support the spine, reducing the pressure on any single disc and reducing the risk of injury.

Hinge at the Hip, Don't Bend in the Back.

To teach yourself to hinge at the hip instead of bending in the back, grab a broom or something similar. Stand up straight with the broom resting down your back. This will help you see your natural alignment, with the shoulders above the chest, the chest above the navel, the navel above the hips. A nice straight line.

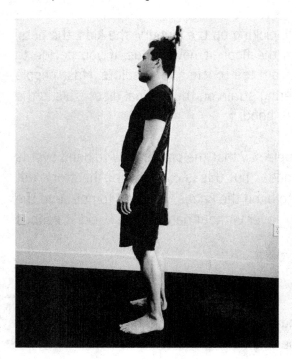 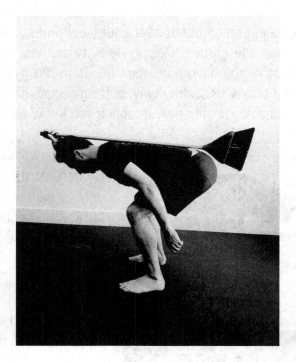

Now hinge at the hip, lowering your torso without bending in the back.

If you have any space between the broom and your back, you're doing it wrong.

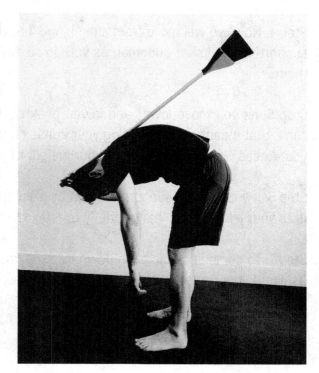

Keeping the spine in the neutral straight position is the proper way to lower and raise the torso towards the ground. You want to maintain the natural alignment of the spine all the way down. The spine isn't meant to bend excessively. It puts too much pressure on the vertebrae when you tilt or bend. Hinging at the hip is the correct way to bend.

With healthy bending habits, you get free exercise hundreds of times a day; strengthen your legs; stop knee pain; and let your discs heal, all at the same time. Hip Hinging will change your life and keep your back happy for a long time to come.

When practicing the TheraQi sequence, we hinge at the hip and then move into a hang. The hang is a type of very gentle inversion. An inversion is a movement or pose where you're upside down. Inversions are popular in yoga because they stimulate the body's systems of health.

Step By Step

Step 1: Stand in the Starting Position, with feet side by side, comfortably apart.

Step 2: Bend both knees. Keep both heels flat, touching the floor.

Step 3: As you bend, keep your upper body upright, as if you don't want something to fall out of your shirt pocket. This will encourage you to hinge at the hip instead of bending in the back.

If you have the strength, stick out your arms overhead to intensify the hinge.

Step 4: Now we will move from a hip hinge into a hang. Slowly "drape" your spine over the thighs, supporting the lower abdomen as you do so. Only bend the back once it's fully supported by the thighs.

Step 5: As you move lower and lower, peek down and make sure you can see your toes. If you can't, that means you are letting your knees come forward too much, which shifts your weight to your knees. You want to ground your weight in your heels, not your knees.

Step 6: If you need to support yourself by placing the hands on the ground, that's okay. Otherwise, grab your elbows and "hang" briefly to relax the spine.

Step 7: To come back up, push down into the ground with the heels, and slowly raise yourself up, "peeling" your upper body away from the thighs, so that your abdomen stays in contact with the thighs for as long as possible. This ensures the lower back is supported for the longest time possible. Keep the knees bent until you have fully raised yourself back up. Push the heels down into the floor for support as you rise.

If you have a history of back pain, or are generally inflexible, you may want to sit in a chair and practice draping the spine over the thighs to stretch the back out. This will ensure your spine is fully supported until you feel comfortable performing the movement standing up.

MOVEMENT INFORMATION

Movement Name
Hip Hinge and Hang

Difficulty
Level 1

Where you'll see it
Physical therapy
Weightlifting - deadlift
What it wakes up
Hips
Back

Contraindications and Cautions
If not performed carefully this can be a dangerous movement, causing damage to the spine. Move slowly and intentionally at all times, keeping the head stable.
If you have any type of back or neck pain or injury, do not perform this movement without the supervision and permission of a doctor.
Move slowly. At no time should you feel any pain or discomfort.

Deepen the Movement
Extend the amount of time you are comfortable being inverted.

In the Beginning...
Do the Broom Test
Have a friend help you check your form

Additional Research
Search: "Hip Hinge"
Search: "Broom Test Hip Hinge"

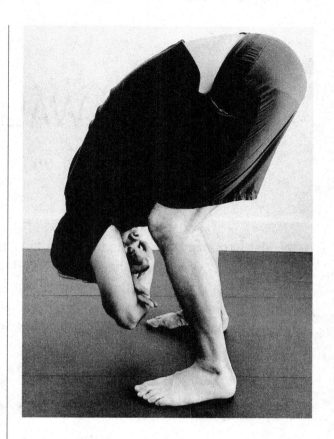

12. WALK-OUTS

Bend over and wiggle your hips.

In the last movement, we learned to hinge the hip as a means of bending over in a safe and supported manner. Once we are hanging upside down, there may be some residual tension in the lower back. The Walk-Out is the next step after a bend. In this movement, we follow up a bend by placing the hands on the ground and wiggling the hips. In doing so, we release any remaining tension in the lower back, hips, hamstrings, and knees.

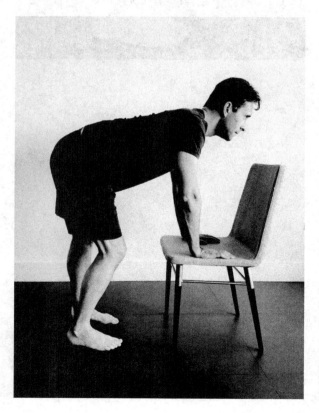

Step By Step

Step 1: Do a hinge and bend, resting the hands on the floor in front of you or on a chair, if that makes you more comfortable.

Step 2: Move the knees back and forth to wiggle your hips, as if you're walking in place.

MOVEMENT INFORMATION

Movement Name
Walk-outs

Difficulty
Level 2

Where you'll see it
Yoga
What it wakes up
Hamstrings
Lower back

Contraindications and Cautions
If not performed carefully this can be a dangerous movement, causing damage to the spine. Move slowly and intentionally at all times, keeping the head stable.
If you have any type of back or neck pain or injury, do not perform this movement without the supervision and permission of a doctor. Move slowly. At no time should you feel any pain or discomfort.

Deepen the Movement
The more you move the knees (bending one while straightening the other) the more intense the stretch will be in the hamstring and back.

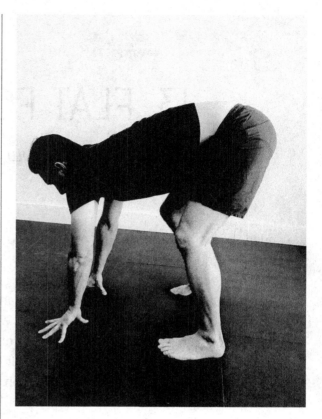

In the Beginning...
If you can't bend all the way over, rest your arms on a chair instead of the floor.
If you find you really struggle, sit in a chair and bend over, with the lap supporting the back. Then wiggle your butt in the chair to loosen the back.

Additional Research
None suggested.

13. FLAT FOOT SQUAT

Squat down with your heels flat on the floor.

We ended the last movement bent over, with our hands on the floor, wiggling our butt. It's time to lower the butt down into a Flat Foot Squat.

The Flat Foot Squat, or Asian Squat, is self-explanatory: it's a squat where the feet stay flat on the ground. This pose is popular in Asian cultures, where you might see someone squatting casually on a sidewalk reading a newspaper or talking on a phone. It's almost impossible for a Westerner to do this pose successfully on the first try. Our bodies just aren't used to it. It can takes months of practice to get it right, so if you struggle, don't take it personally. This is a challenging move.

I like performing the Flat Foot Squat because it increases balance and flexibility while strengthening the core considerably. Also, if you can pull it off, you'll impress your friends at parties.

What exactly is a squat? A squat happens when there is maximal bending (smallest angle) at the knees and the waist. A bend happens when there is minimal bending of the knees and maximal bending of the waist only. When you bend over, you bend at the waist keeping the legs mostly straight. If you bend over, and then bend the knees also, you end up in a squat.

In the previous movements, you learned to hinge the hip at the waist and bend over. Remember that the Hip Hinge is about reducing the angle between the thigh and the abdomen to the smallest angle possible. Once you are in that position (bent over at the waist) bend the knees as well to lower the butt down to the floor, keeping the heels flat on the floor. The Flat Foot Squat is a next natural move from the Hip Hinge and Hang.

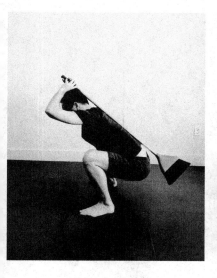 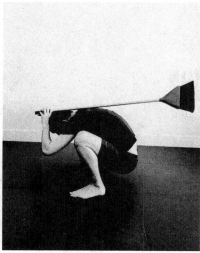

When practicing the move, use your broom to help you determine if you're keeping the spine straight, and not rounded. In the beginning you will be rounded. Just keep practicing.

The range of motion this pose creates in the lower body is impressive to experience. When you master it you'll feel invincible.

Step By Step

Step 1: Stand in Starting Position.

Step 2: Follow the steps for the Hip Hinge and Hang. Bend the knees slightly, and drape the spine over the thighs until your hands touch the floor.

Step 3: Do a Walk-Out wiggle to loosen any tension in the knees and lower back.

Step 4: Shift your weight to the heels, and slowly drop the butt to the floor by bending the knees.

Step 5: Lower your sit bones all the way down to just a few inches off the floor and balance yourself, keeping the feet flat. Lift your arms up overhead to deepen the movement.

Step 6: To come up, reverse the movement. Push yourself up via the heels and straighten the knees so that you are back in the Hang/Walk-out position. Then slowly lift yourself up like you would in the Hip Hinge and Hang, carefully peeling your spine off the thighs, until you return to Starting Position.

MOVEMENT INFORMATION

Movement Name
Flat Foot Squat; Asian Squat

Difficulty
Level 3

Where you'll see it
Asian street corners

What it wakes up
Hips and butt
Lower back
Hamstrings
Knees

Contraindications and Cautions
This movement can put strain on the lower back and the knees, so if you're not flexible, don't try to go down all the way. You must make sure you're ready for the intensity of this stretch.

Deepen the Movement
Perfect the form by keeping the back straight. Learn to hold the pose for a longer period of time.

In the Beginning...
Don't be ashamed to hold on to something to keep your balance.

Additional Research

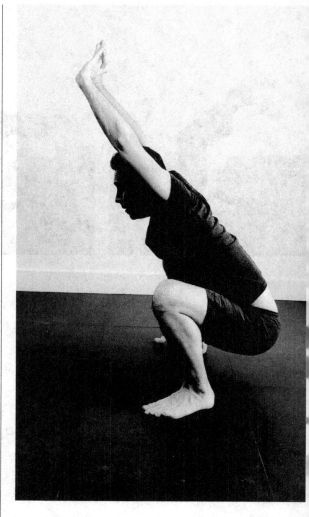

Search: "How to Asian Squat" or "Flat Foot Squat"
Search: "How to Hindu Squat"

14. DOWNWARD DOG

Do your version of a Downward Dog.

When doing the Flat Foot Squat, you can also easily move into a Downward Dog, a popular yoga position that stretches and strengthens the entire body.

Yoga for me has always been love/hate. I've tried practicing yoga over the years to mixed results. I started with Richard Hittleman's "Yoga in 28 Days" book back in the 1980's, and eventually stumbled into several Iyengar Yoga classrooms before finally giving up after a particularly challenging Bikram class. I struggle with yoga. I find yoga boring, painful, and difficult. Despite my distaste for it, I do have one move I love: the (heavily modified) Downward Dog.

The Downward Dog offers a complete full body stretch, from the tops of the fingers down to the tips of the toes. It is a simple but powerful movement that is difficult to master. Despite my dislike of yoga, I do a version of Downward Dog everyday as part of my daily TheraQi practice to keep my legs limber and my lower back free of pain.

The heart of the Downward Dog is the Hip Hinge. The Downward Dog is basically an inverted Hip Hinge, with the hands and feet on the ground. Instead of closing the hinge, the hands and feet are anchored so that the hinge can't close. This causes the pelvis to push upward, away from the hands and feet, stretching and elongating the arms, legs, and back. It's like pulling back on a slingshot.

Doing a proper Downward Dog is challenging. The hands are feet are on the floor, and the weight of the body is supported by the hands. The heels go down to the ground, and wow, does it burn.

Over the years, I've discovered a few modifications to the Downward Dog that are easier for my locked up body to perform. I share them with you so that you may find a version of this wonderful move that is suitable for your level of strength and flexibility (and maybe your pain tolerance too). Choose whatever version of the movement you feel most comfortable with. Just promise yourself you'll practice it every day.

Step By Step

Classical Downward Dog:

This is the hardest version. Level 3.

Step 1: Begin on your hands and knees. Align your wrists directly under your shoulders with your knees directly under your hips so you're sort of curled up underneath yourself.

Step 2: Pop yourself up into the shape of an inverted V, with fingers spread wide and your toes planted on the floor.

Step 3: Push the pelvis up towards the ceiling and point the sit bones towards the wall behind you.

Step 4: Push the heels down into the floor as you lift your pelvis up. This will give you an intense stretch.

Step 5: Push your hands down into the ground and squeeze the elbows so they are just behind the ears (like in the overhead stretch).

Step 6: Hold as long as you can and come down.

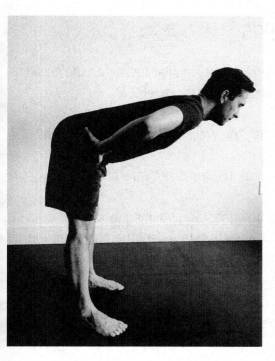

Standing Downward Dog:

This version is very easy to do, and can be done most anywhere with or without a chair for support. It is not as beneficial as some of the other versions, however, so I would only use it as a stepping stone to the other versions. Level 1.

Step 1: Stand up straight and with the hands on the hips.

Step 2: Keeping the back straight and the chest pushed out, hinge at the hip without bending the knees.

Step 3: Slowly lower the straightened torso towards the floor without bending the knees. It's as though you're trying to keep something from falling out of your shirt pocket.

Step 4: Only go down as far as you can without bending the back or knees. The ideal will be to get to a 90 degree angle, but you may only get to 45.

If this movement is difficult, place a chair in front of you, and rest your hands on the seat of the chair. Push down into the seat with your hands while pushing into the floor with the heels. Keep the back and legs straight.

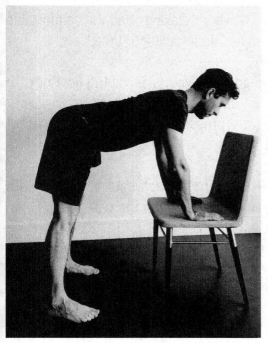

Standing Wall-Supported Downward Dog

This version is by far my favorite. It's easy to do, and provides a very similar feeling as the classical version, only it doesn't put as much pressure on the arms and wrists. Level 2.

Step 1: Stand in front of a wall with your hands flat against the wall, right at shoulder height.

Step 2: Keeping the hands on the wall, walk backwards until the arms are stretched out.

Step 3: Drop the torso while pushing into the wall with the hands and pushing into the floor with the heels. Push the sit bones up and out. As the pelvis pushes outward, feel the pull on the arms and legs. It will feel like you are "hanging" from the wall with your palms. You should feel a deep stretch in the arms, legs, and lower back.

Lying Wall-Supported Downward Dog

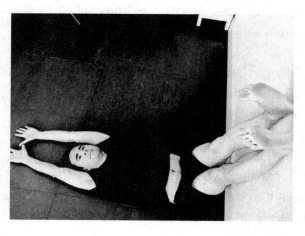

This one is very relaxing, and is comfortable enough to be held for a longer time. Level 1.

Step 1: Lie down on your side, on the floor next to a wall. Curl up and wiggle yourself so that your sit bones are pressed against the baseboard of the wall.

Step 2: Slowly turn yourself onto your back with your legs loosely resting on the wall.

Step 3: Push the backs of the heels against the wall, straightening the legs until the knees are locked. Reach your arms overhead onto the floor. Ideally you would be able to make a 90 degree angle. If you're not flexible enough, you might need to push yourself out farther from the wall.

MOVEMENT INFORMATION

Movement Name
Downward Dog

Difficulty
Level 1 (Standing Downward Dog)
Level 2 (Lying Downward Dog)
Level 3 (Classic Downward Dog)
Where you'll see it
Yoga

What it wakes up
Hamstrings
Arms, wrists, hands
Back, shoulders, and shoulder girdle

Contraindications and Cautions
If you have any type of back or neck pain or injury, do not perform this movement without the supervision and permission of a doctor. Move slowly. At no time should you feel any pain or discomfort.

Deepen the Movement
Daily practice.

In the Beginning...
Don't overstretch the hamstrings.
Don't be afraid to start out with easier versions.
If you are very inflexible, do a standing Downward Dog and rest your palms on a chair in front of you.

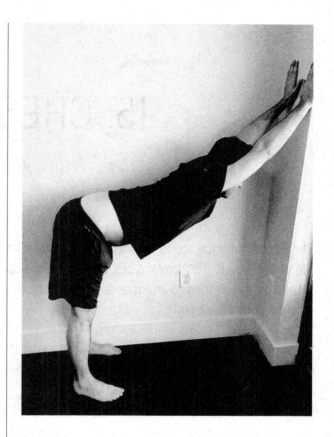

Additional Research
Search: "Downward Dog" and "Downward Dog Modifications"

15. CHEST HULA

Hula your chest.

The TheraQi sequence is intentionally created to provide a natural ebb and flow of intensity. The Flat Foot Squat and Downward Dog are physically demanding. Now it's time for something less intense. Let's return to isolations and pick up where we left off before the inversion exercises. We turn now to Chest Hula.

Chest Hula is a movement to isolate and expand the range of motion of the chest. Imagine having a Hula hoop around your chest and trying to keep it going. That's Chest Hula.

If you have trouble getting the hang of the movement, focus first on getting comfortable with the endpoints of the movement. You did the same thing with Head Hula. Practice thrusting the nipple-line forward and then pulling it back as far as you can. Do that movement a few times and then try to master sliding the nipple-line to the right and left side without tilting or turning. When you've got your four endpoints covered, then try to connect them with a circular motion.

Chest Hula greatly expands the range of motion of the chest, giving you a more youthful, flexible spine.

Step By Step

Step 1: Stick out the chest and arch the back.

Step 2: Keeping the nipple-line parallel to the floor (with no tilting or turning) slide the chest to the right side in a circular fashion.

Step 3: Slide the nipple-line backwards so that your chest is collapsed and the upper back is thrust outward.

Step 4: Continuing the circular motion, slide to the left side.

Step 5: Return to the forward position of Step 1.

Repeat several times until the motion becomes smooth, then repeat in the opposite direction.

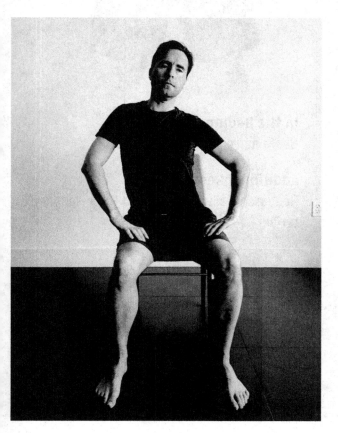

MOVEMENT INFORMATION

Movement Name
Chest Hula

Difficulty
Level 3

Where you'll see it
Hula Hooping
Jazz dance

What it wakes up
Spine
Chest
Abdominals

Contraindications and Cautions
If not performed carefully this can be a dangerous movement, causing damage to the spine. Move slowly and intentionally at all times, keeping the head stable.
If you have any type of back or neck pain or injury, do not perform this movement without the supervision and permission of a doctor.
Move slowly. At no time should you feel any pain or discomfort.
Do not over-extend. Small is better.

Deepen the Movement
Do your best to prevent the chest from tilting. The more you can keep the nipple line parallel to the floor, the deeper the movement will be.

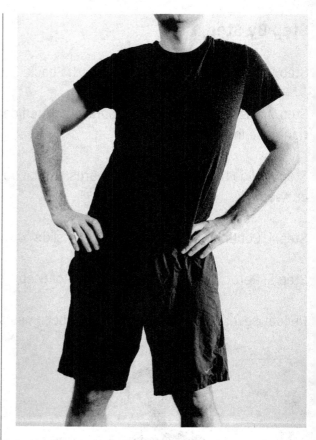

In the Beginning...
Use a mirror to check your form.

Additional Research
Research Belly Dancing and Hula Hooping tutorials.

16. PELVIS HULA

Hula your pelvis.

Continuing the Hula motion down the body, it's time to Hula the Pelvis. The movement after this one is the Hip Hula. The difference between the Hip Hula and the Pelvis Hula is that the Pelvis Hula is a smaller, tighter movement in which the pelvis "circle-slides" around the spine. It's a true isolation in which the rest of the body stays very still. The Hip Hula is not a pure isolation. It's more of a circular hinge at the hip with the spine staying relatively straight. The Pelvis Hula is exclusively focused on manipulating the pelvis to stretch and expand the range of motion of the lower spine.

As with other forms of Hula, if you have trouble getting the hang of the movement, focus first on getting the endpoints of the movement. Practice thrusting the pelvis forward (tucking it under the torso) and then pulling it back as far as you can (but keep the sit bones pointing down, not up). Do that movement a few times and then try to master the right and left slide. When you've got your four endpoints covered, then try to connect them with a sliding circle motion.

Step By Step

Step 1: Stand up straight and thrust the pelvis forward, tucking it under your torso.

Step 2: Keeping the pelvis level (parallel to the floor, without tilting or turning) slide the pelvis to the right side.

Step 3: Slide the pelvis backwards so that the back is very flat. Don't stick the sit bones up and out, point them down into the ground.

Step 4: Keeping the pelvis level, slide it to the left side.

Step 5: Slide back to the front as you did in Step 1.

Repeat several times until the motion becomes smooth, then repeat in the opposite direction.

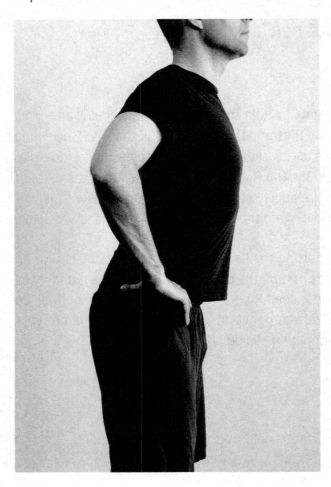

MOVEMENT INFORMATION

Movement Name
Pelvis Hula

Difficulty
Level 3

Where you'll see it
Hula hooping
Ballet

What it wakes up
Abdominals
Lower back
Butt

Contraindications and Cautions
If not performed carefully this can be a dangerous movement, causing damage to the neck and spine. Move slowly and intentionally at all times, keeping the head stable.
If you have any type of neck pain or injury, do not perform this movement without the supervision and permission of a doctor.
Move slowly. At no time should you feel any pain or discomfort.
Do not over-extend. Small is better.

Deepen the Movement
Practice the movement with different ranges of motion and for longer periods of time.

In the Beginning...
Use a mirror to check your form.

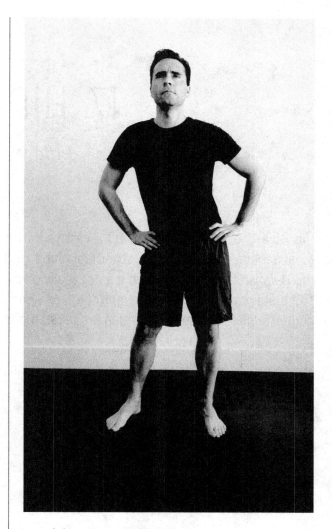

Additional Research
None suggested.

17. HIP HULA

Hula your hips.

Hip Hula is a more relaxed, playful version of the Hula than we've seen before. The other Hulas (head, chest, and pelvis) are strict isolations, and if performed carelessly can hurt the spine. The Hip Hula isn't an isolation and it's not really about the spine at all. The knees are slightly bent, the spine stays nice and straight, and the hips open to hinge the hips in a big circle. It's a safe, easy, comfortable movement that releases tension and just feels fun.

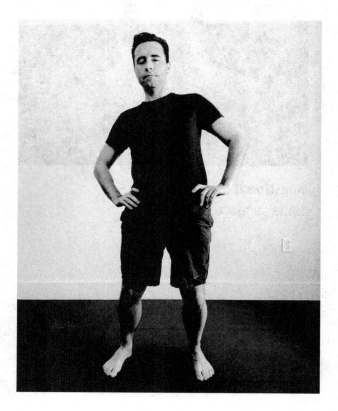

Step By Step

Step 1: Stand up straight and thrust the hips forward. Keep the legs mostly straight. A slight bend is fine. Be sure to keep the feet flat on the floor.

Step 2: Move the hips in a big circle clockwise, then counterclockwise.

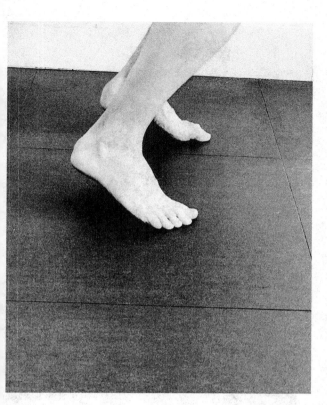

Step 3: After moving in both directions, repeat the motion, but this time allow your feet to rock back and forth so that the weight of your body shifts from the ball of the foot to the heel. When the hips are thrust forward, shift your weight to the balls of the feet, and lift the heels off the ground. When you swing the hips around behind you, shift your weight to the heels, lifting the toes and balls of the feet off the floor. As you move the hips in a circle, rock your body back and forth on the feet.

Repeat both styles (flat foot and rocked feet) several times until the motion becomes smooth, then repeat in the opposite direction.

MOVEMENT INFORMATION

Movement Name
Hip Hula

Difficulty
Level 1

Where you'll see it
Hula hooping
Jazz isolations
Pilates

What it wakes up
Hip joints
Abdominals
Leg muscles

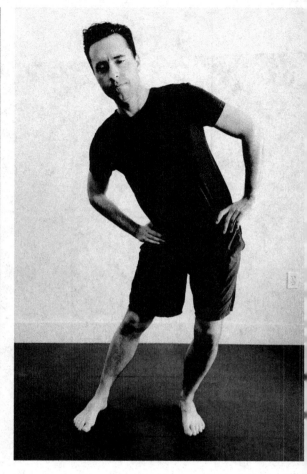

Contraindications and Cautions
If not performed carefully this can be a dangerous movement, causing damage to the spine. Move slowly and intentionally at all times.
If you have any type of back or neck pain or injury, do not perform this movement without the supervision and permission of a doctor.
Move slowly. At no time should you feel any pain or discomfort.

Deepen the Movement
Alternate between Hip Hula and Pelvis Hula to explore the differences between the motions.

In the Beginning...
If you can't get the hang of the "rocking" of the weight from ball to heel with the Hip Hula, try standing straight and rocking back and forth on your feet without the circles, to get the hang of the motion. Once you feel comfortable rocking back and forth, then try to add in the hip circles.

Additional Research
Search: "Pelvic Circles" or "Hip Circles"

18. TIP TOE SQUAT

Squat down on your tip toes.

In the last movement, we practiced shifting the weight of the body onto the balls of the feet and then the heels. This movement, the Tip Toe Squat, builds on that motion by shifting the weight of the body to the balls of the feet, and then lowering the torso down towards the ground by deeply bending the knees.

Being able to squat down and stand up again is an important marker of a youthful body. Squatting is a foundation of strength and fitness. This particular squat opens the knees and leg muscles and stretches the muscles of the hips and pelvis area.

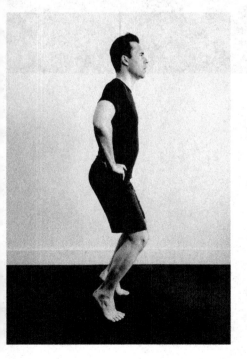

Step By Step

Step 1: Standing in Starting Position, shift the weight of the body to the balls of the feet, lifting the heels. In other words, stand on your toes.

Step 2: Slowly lower the body down to the floor, keeping the heels lifted off the ground.

Step 3: Straighten the back so that you stand on your toes nice and tall. Do your best to keep your balance.

MOVEMENT INFORMATION

Movement Name
Tip Toe Squat

Difficulty
Level 3

Where you'll see it
The Awkward Pose in yoga.

What it wakes up
Legs, toes, feet, ankles

Contraindications and Cautions
If you have any ankle or knee problems, be extra careful.

Deepen the Movement
Practice holding the pose for longer periods of time.

In the Beginning...
Use your hands to help keep your balance.

Additional Research
Search: "Awkward Pose" or "Tip Toe Squat"

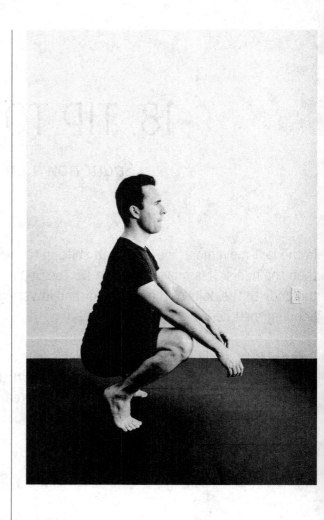

19. DOUBLE HULA

Hula your chest and hips at the same time.

Earlier in the sequence, you learned to do various isolation movements, including the chest, hips, head/neck, and pelvis. When we introduced the idea of isolations, we said that these movements can be combined to form complex motions in which two or more isolated movements are happening at the same time.

A simple explanation of this would be to pat the head and rub the tummy at the same time. Neither movement has anything to do with the other, but if you're coordinated enough you can find a way to make the rhythm of the two movements align so that it's one motion.

The Double Hula is a combined isolation movement. The Double Hula is a combination of the Pelvis Hula and the Chest Hula. In this motion, the chest and pelvis both move in the same direction, but they are moving at opposite ends, much like the knees did in the Figure 8. When the chest slides to the right, the pelvis slides to the left. When the pelvis slides forward, the chest slides back.

The real opportunity of this movement is to increase your coordination, and to discover how different parts of the body are connected. When first learning this movement, you might think of it as two distinct motions: moving the chest and moving the pelvis. After you get the hang of it, you'll see that the chest and pelvis are intimately connected and the rotation of one causes the rotation of the other. In the same way that alternately bending and straightening the knees can cause the hips to wiggle, the movement of the pelvis causes the movement of the chest, and vice versa. It's very satisfying to experience the connectedness of your body.

Still, this is a very challenging movement and can take weeks if not months of practice. Don't get discouraged. Use a mirror and keep trying until you get your body to do what your brain tells it to do.

Joseph Pilates said, "If your spine is inflexibly stiff at 30, you are old; if it is completely flexible at 60, you are young." This movement is a diagnostic for the vitality of your spine.

Step By Step

Step 1: Do a few Pelvis Hulas to warm yourself up, then bring your attention to your chest. Discover how the movement of the hips can drive the movement of the chest in the opposite direction.

Step 2: Stop the movement and instead do the chest Hula, and bring your attention to the pelvis. Discover how the motion of the chest can drive the motion of the pelvis in the opposite direction.

Step 3: Keep practicing until you can experience the opposing motions of the chest and pelvis as one single motion, two entities moving as one, smoothly and effortlessly.

MOVEMENT INFORMATION

Movement Name
Double Hula

Difficulty
Level 3

Where you'll see it
Belly dancing
Pilates
Jazz dance
What it wakes up
Spine
Abdominals
Back muscles

Contraindications and Cautions
If not performed carefully this can be a dangerous movement, causing damage to the neck and spine. Move slowly and intentionally at all times, keeping the head stable.
If you have any type of neck pain or injury, do not perform this movement without the supervision and permission of a doctor.
Move slowly. At no time should you feel any pain or discomfort.
Do not over-extend. Small is better.

Deepen the Movement
Take it to the next level by adding the head to create a Triple Hula. The head will align with the pelvis, and the chest will move in opposition. This is a major achievement of coordination.

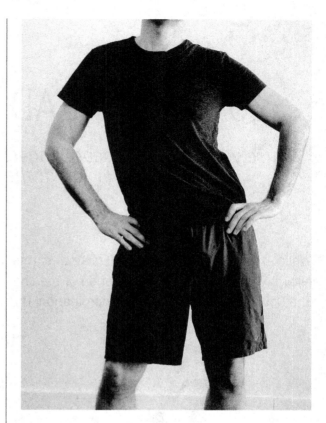

In the Beginning...
Use a mirror to check your form.
Be patient.
Master the individual isolations (Chest Hula and Pelvis Hula) first.

Additional Research
None suggested.

20. OVERHEAD DOUBLE HULA

Raise your arms overhead, fingers clasped, and hula your hips and chest at the same time.

While executing the Double Hula, raise the arms overhead into Overhead Stretch. Adding the arms allows you to exaggerate the motion of the chest, deepening the stretch in the ribcage and back. The Double Stretch is a feat of coordination; this movement just feels good.

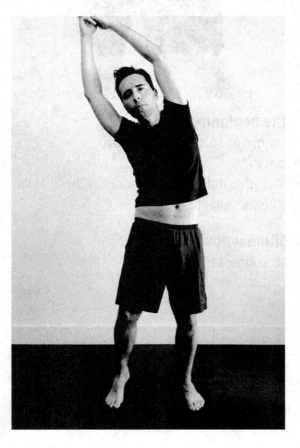

Step By Step

Step 1: Do the Double Hula.

Step 2: Lift the arms up into the Overhead Stretch, fingers interlaced and palms together.

Step 3: Use the exaggeration of the arms to further elongate and exaggerate the motion of the chest, which will in turn help separate the motion of the chest from that of the hips.

MOVEMENT INFORMATION

Movement Name
Overhead Double Hula

Difficulty
Level 3

Where you'll see it
Dance
Pilates

What it wakes up
Chest
Arms

Contraindications and Cautions
If not performed carefully this can be a dangerous movement, causing damage to the neck and spine. Move slowly and intentionally at all times, keeping the head stable.
If you have any type of neck pain or injury, do not perform this movement without the supervision and permission of a doctor.
Move slowly. At no time should you feel any pain or discomfort.
Do not over-extend. Small is better.

Deepen the Movement
Execute the Double Hula while hanging from a pull-up bar. The arms remain stationary, and the chest and pelvis move in the opposite directions.

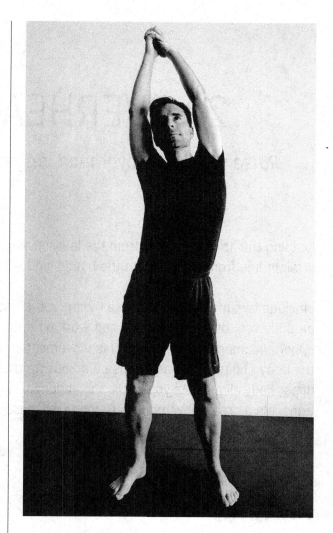

In the Beginning...
Use a mirror to check your form.

Additional Research
None suggested.

21. OVERHEAD HIP HULA

Raise your arms overhead, fingers clasped, and hula your hips.

Keeping the arms overhead from the last movement, stop the movement of the chest to create a straight line from the pelvis to the hands, and shift into a hip Hula.

I include this movement because I want you to discover how subtle changes to a movement can produce very different feelings and work different muscles. The Overhead Double Hula works the upper abdomen and the chest. This movement extends the center of gravity beyond the midline of the body and provides an intense workout for the abdominals. It is physically difficult to keep the upper body aligned. As you circle, the abdominals have to work overtime to stabilize the overhead arms. It's a great movement to toughen up those abdominals.

Additionally, I love the way this movement removes all the tension from the muscles of the lower back and sides.

Step By Step

Follow the instructions for the Hip Hula, and bring the arms overhead, fingers interlaced, palms together. Feel the exaggeration of the movement and enjoy the stretching it provides.

MOVEMENT INFORMATION

Movement Name
Overhead Hip Hula

Difficulty
Level 1

Where you'll see it
Belly Dancing

What it wakes up
Lower back
Chest
Arms
Abdomen

Contraindications and Cautions
Raising the arms overhead in this movement can shift your center of gravity, placing extra strain on the lower back as you Hula. Be especially careful as you widen the movement, being sure that your abdomen is firmly supporting the back and you are not extending beyond your comfort zone.
If you have any type of neck pain or injury, do not perform this movement without the supervision and permission of a doctor.
Move slowly. At no time should you feel any pain or discomfort.

Deepen the Movement
Execute this movement while hanging from a pull-up bar. The arms remain stationary, and the pelvis moves in an exaggerated Hula motion.

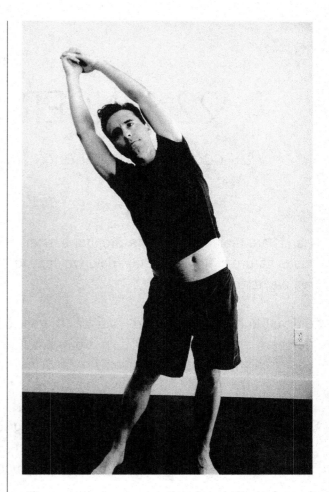

Alternate between an Overhead Hip Hula and an Overhead Pelvis Hula. The movement is essentially the same but the shift between the pelvis and the hips will provide different sensations.

In the Beginning…
Use a mirror to check your form.

Additional Research
None suggested.

22. FINGER STRETCHES

Pull back and stretch each finger and thumb, one at a time.

Hands are remarkable things. Stop for a moment and look at your hand. Be present to the miraculous nature of its complexity. How we depend on these little machines, and how little attention we pay to them.

Did you know that there are over 27 different bones in the human hand and over 34 muscles? Compare that to the arm, which has only 3 bones and 23 muscles. If we were to dole out exercise based on the quantity and quality of muscles, bones, and joints, we could quickly see that the hands do not get the fitness love that they deserve.

Over the next several movements, you're going to discover a new relationship to your hands by getting to know the way they move and work in a fundamentally deeper way. You'll never see your hands with same sleepy eyes again. The gratitude will radiate from your heart.

The first of these movements is the Finger Stretch. Simply pull back gently on each finger individually to stretch the hand, finger, and wrist. This movement will release tension in the hands and strengthen the fingers. It also is great for increasing the range of motion of the fingers, wrists, and palm.

Step By Step

Finger Stretches are best performed with the arm fully extended and the elbow locked. This will ensure the deepest stretch possible.

Step 1: Extend the left arm and lock the elbow. Using the right hand, pull back gently on the left little finger. Keep the other fingers relaxed. If you like, you can massage the finger gently with the right hand, and/or wiggle it gently. If you do, just don't lose sight of the original intention: to pull back gently on the finger to give it a stretch. Hold the stretch for as long as you feel comfortable and not more.

Step 2: Repeat the above step for the remaining fingers of both hands.

Step 3: After stretching all your fingers individually, stretch the four fingers of each hand together. You can practice this pose by pressing the palm into a wall, fingers down and forearm up.

MOVEMENT INFORMATION

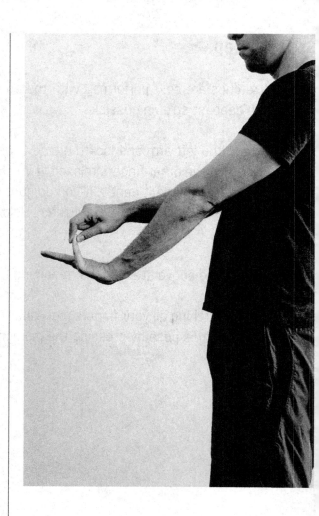

Movement Name
Finger Stretches

Difficulty
Level 1

Where you'll see it
Physical therapy

What it Wakes Up
Fingers, thumbs, palms, wrists
Forearms

Contraindications and Cautions
If you have carpal tunnel syndrome or other injuries of the hands or wrists, be particularly careful. Over-stretching can be dangerous.

Deepen the Movement
You can deepen this movement by resisting the stretch, pushing against the pulling hand with the finger being pulled. After resisting, relax again. Alternating this resist/relax movement will deepen the stretch and further strengthen the arm and hand.

In the Beginning...
Be gentle.

Additional Research
Search: "Finger Stretches"

23. FINGER CIRCLES

Circumduct each finger and thumb.

My personal mission, and the purpose of creating the TheraQi sequence, is to educate people about how the human body moves, so that they can use movement to live happier and healthier lives. So far, we've learned about Hula and isolations. For example, in Chapter 5, I described the movement of the head and neck, and how the joints in the neck can tilt on an angle, turn from side to side, or slide over the top of one another. This brings awareness to the body where it was lacking.

I also explored pushing weight away from the body and pulling weight towards the body.

Now I want to introduce another big theme in movement that's based on circles. Besides flexing and extending, the elbow, miracle that it is, can move 360 degrees, not just back and forth like in a bicep curl. By moving the elbow in its full range of motion, we can trace a cone-like shape: the point of the cone is the elbow, and the open point of the cone is where the hand makes a circle at the other end.

There is a little-known scientific word for this motion: circumduction. What a mouthful. It's a silly word for a wonderful motion. Circumduction engages the full range of the body's movement. It's a fast, efficient, and enjoyable way to move the body, opening the body and expanding the range of motion. What makes circumduction distinct from just "making a circle" with a body part, is that circumduction only happens when a body part is fixed on one end and open on the other.

With Hula we made circles with the pelvis and chest. But those don't make cone-like shapes; they are fixed at both ends. Hula and circumduction both make circles, but only one of them makes a cone, and that's only possible with certain body parts.

The foot can be circumducted from the fixed point of the ankle; the lower part of the arm can be circumducted from the elbow; the entire arm circumducted from the shoulder, etc. The eyes circumduct, because they are attached to the body at one end and not the other.

Circumduction matters because it engages the entire possible expression of the body. Flexing and extending force the body to move in rigid, fixed, limited ways. Circumduction is literally the freedom to unleash the body in any direction. It's a radically different way of thinking about and moving the body.

TheraQi could easily be called "The Circumduction Workout," there's so much of it. The sequence will have you circumduct the fingers, hands/wrist, elbows/arms, shoulders/arms, feet/ankles, lower leg/knees, thighs/hips and the eyes.

Circular motion (both circumduction and the hula-style circular joint slides) forms the foundation of TheraQi. Circular motion moves the body past the rigid back and forth of flexing and extending, movements that are repetitive and boring. Your body has so much potential to move, and circular motion unlocks that potential, extending your range of movement, lubricating your joints, and making movement more pleasurable and fun.

Finger Circles

Once you understand the concept of the circumduction cone-shape, it's easy to circumduct a body part. In the Finger Circles movement, we make circles with all our individual fingers, which stretches out the individual fingers and improves dexterity and hand strength.

As you do this motion, you'll notice that some fingers are easier than others. The thumb and index finger are easy, but the other fingers are a bit harder to move. And you may find your dominant hand (for most people, the right hand) easier than the non-dominant hand. As a right-handed person, I struggle to perform this movement with my left ring-finger. You don't have to obsess on the form, the important thing is to engage the brain and try to do your best.

Step By Step

Step 1: Hold the right hand flat in front of you, palms down, with your thumb extended away from the hand.

Step 2: Circumduct your thumb, making as big and wide a circle as you can. Keep the other fingers still.

Step 3: Reverse the direction of the circumduction.

Step 4: Repeat Steps 2 and 3 with the remaining fingers on both hands.

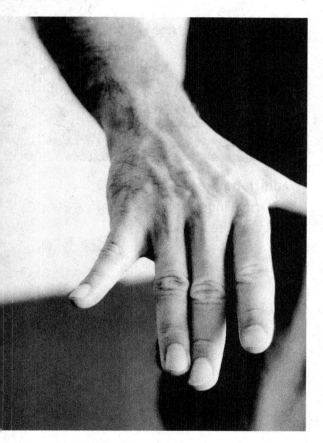

MOVEMENT INFORMATION

Movement Name
Finger Circles

Difficulty
Level 2

Where you'll see it
Physical therapy
Qigong

What it Wakes Up
Fingers, thumbs, wrists, palms
Forearms

Contraindications and Cautions
If you have carpal tunnel syndrome or other injuries of the hands or wrists, be particularly careful. Over-stretching can be dangerous.

Deepen the Movement
Explore the entire range of motion. When raising the hand up, feel the back of the hand pull towards the top of the forearm, making as close to a 90 degree angle as you can. It will look like a "stop sign" with the palm extended. Do the same on the downward motion, with the palm making a 90 degree angle with the underside of the forearm when the fingers are pointed to the floor.

In the Beginning...
Imagine your finger is a laser pointer. Draw imaginary laser circles on the wall.

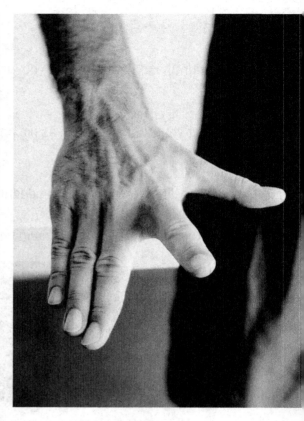

Additional Research
Search: "Finger Circumduction"
Search: "Circumduction"

24. FINGER WAVES

Wiggle your fingers.

In the last exercise, we started to distinguish the movement of each finger in isolation from the others by circumducting each finger individually. In Finger Waves, we move the fingers in a wave. By wave, I don't mean pumping the fingers up and down together like a princess waving at her prince. I mean moving them one at a time, like audience members doing the wave in a stadium.

The easiest way to experience this motion is to simply wiggle your fingers. More than likely, you'll wiggle them in a wave. You can also learn the motion by tapping the fingers on a table, as if you're impatient. The rapid rise and fall of the fingers against the table top will make a sound like a galloping horse.

Once you grasp the idea of the finger wave, add a figure eight motion to the hand while the fingers wave independently. The combination of the fingers and hands moving together makes for a very powerful exercise.

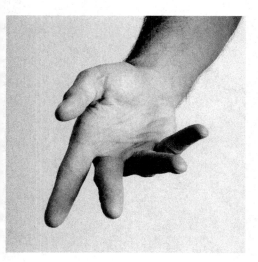

Step By Step

Step 1: Hold the hand in front of you and move the fingers in a wave pattern, including the thumb.

Step 2: Repeat with the other hand.

Step 3: Add a figure eight motion with the wrist to create a more complex movement that intensifies the stretch.

MOVEMENT INFORMATION

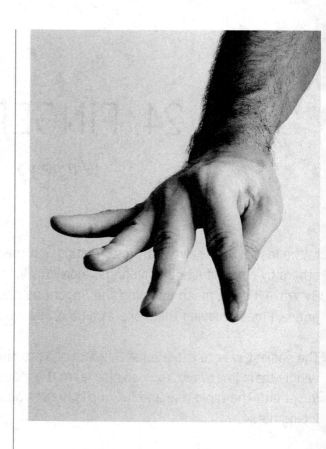

Movement Name
Finger Waves

Difficulty
Level 3

Where you'll see it
Chinese Baoding Balls
Qigong
Tai Chi

What it Wakes Up
Fingers, thumbs, wrists, palms
Forearms

Contraindications and Cautions
If you have carpal tunnel syndrome or other injuries of the hands or wrists, be particularly careful. Over-stretching can be dangerous.

Deepen the Movement
Perform this motion inside a bucket filled with rice.
Combine the finger wave with a figure-eight motion of the wrist.

In the Beginning...
If you struggle with this movement, watch videos of "Chinese Baoding Balls" and notice the movement of the fingers.

Additional Research
Search: "Chinese Baoding Balls"
Search: "Qigong Finger Movement"

25. FINGER CURLS

Repeatedly curl your fingers into a claw.

The previous couple of movements have been very loose. This motion and the next are more tense. In Finger Curls, we flex the fingers. Flexing means the body curls up on itself. In this movement, the fingers are curling up towards the palm to close the hand into something like a fist. The fist we make here is not a regular fist, but a Tiger Claw. A Tiger Claw is made by bending the fingers at the two outer-most knuckles, but not at the base knuckle where the finger attaches to the hand.

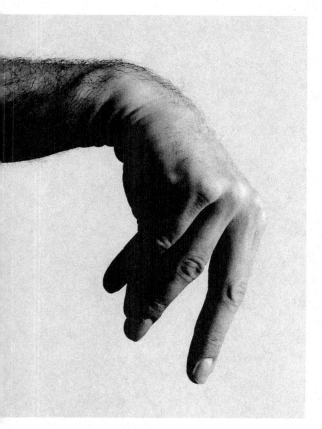

The fingers hang down, and are then pulled up tight into a Tiger Claw.

When this motion becomes fluid, your hand will undulate like a jellyfish floating through the water.

The movement should be flowing and smooth.

This motion, along with its opposite, the Finger Extension, will greatly enhance the strength and dexterity of your hands. These motions will improve your fine motor skills and release tension in the wrist, forearms, fingers, and especially thumbs.

Step By Step

Step 1: Place the hand in front of your body, palm down to the floor, with the fingers slightly extended.

Step 2: Reach down with the fingers and pull up into the palm with all fingers simultaneously Imagine grabbing dough with the hand and squeezing the dough through your fingers.

Step 3: As you pull up the fingers, pull the wrist back so that the top of the hand is in a 90 degree angle to the top of the forearm. As you pull the wrist back, pull the fingers into a tiger claw.

Step 4: Repeat the motion with the other hand.

MOVEMENT INFORMATION

Movement Name
Finger Curls

Difficulty
Level 1

Where you'll see it
Kung Fu Tiger Claw
Tai Chi
Qigong

What it Wakes Up
Fingers, thumbs, wrists, palms
Forearms

Contraindications and Cautions
If you have carpal tunnel syndrome or other injuries of the hands or wrists, be particularly careful. Over-stretching can be dangerous.

Deepen the Movement
Perform this motion inside a bucket filled with rice.

In the Beginning...
If this movement is difficult, simply open and close the hand several times, putting your attention on the closing motion, as though you are squeezing a rubber ball.

Additional Research
Search: "Kung Fu Tiger Claw" to see the hand curl in action.

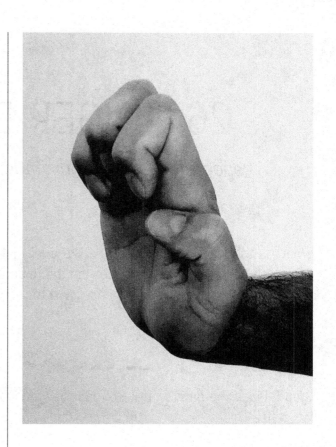

26. FINGER EXTENSIONS

Repeatedly spread your fingers out to look like a starfish.

Whereas the last movement looked like a jellyfish, this movement looks like a starfish. Here, we extend the fingers to open and stretch the fingers and palm. The tendons that control the fingers travel all the way through the hand down to the wrist. This motion gives them a good stretch to keep them young and flexible.

Step By Step

Step 1: Place the hand in front of your body, palm down to the floor, with the fingers curled in a loose fist.

Step 2: Quickly and forcefully open the hand and extend the fingers, doing your best to create as much space between the fingers as you can. It will be like a flick of the hand.

Step 3: Curl the fingers again into a loose fist and repeat Step 2. Repeat this several times.

Step 4: Repeat the above with the opposite hand.

MOVEMENT INFORMATION

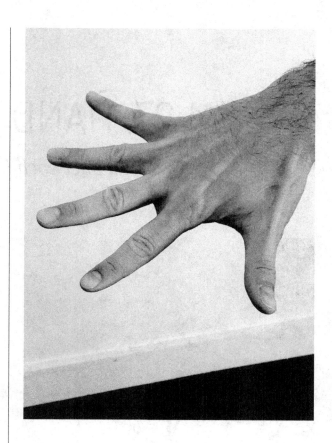

Movement Name
Finger Extensions

Difficulty
Level 1

Where you'll see it
Physical therapy
Qigong

What it Wakes Up
Fingers, thumbs, wrists, palms
Forearms

Contraindications and Cautions
If you have carpal tunnel syndrome or other injuries of the hands or wrists, be particularly careful. Over-stretching can be dangerous.

Deepen the Movement
Perform this motion inside a bucket filled with rice.

In the Beginning...
Focus on spreading the fingers as much as possible.

Additional Research
None suggested.

27. HAND CIRCLES

Circumduct each hand at the wrist.

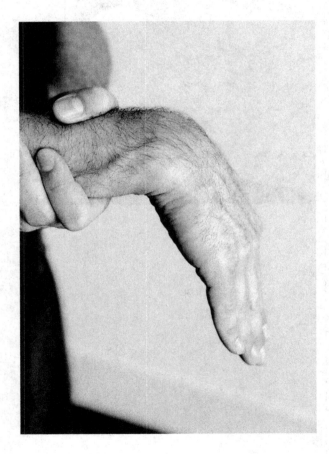

We started the circumduction at the fingers and we will work our way up the arm. It's time to circumduct the hand at the wrist. Stick out your hand and move it in a circle, keeping the forearm still. While circumducting the right hand, hold the right forearm with the left hand to keep the arm from moving.

This seemingly simple move can provide an incredibly strenuous workout for the forearms if you widen the circle as much as possible.

Move the hand intentionally to make the motion count. If you're just letting the hand wobble or wiggle you won't get the benefit. Reach through the motion like you're swimming through peanut butter or quicksand. Extend the range of motion all the way through to open the hand as you move it. Bring the fingers all the way down and all the way up. Make the movement matter

Step By Step

Step 1: Place the hand in front of your body with the palm down towards the floor.

Step 2: Pop the hand up towards the ceiling, making a "Stop" sign with the hand. Feel the stretch in the palm and in the back of the hand.

Step 3: Circumduct the hand, making a big circle in a counterclockwise direction.

Step 4: Repeat this motion several times.

Step 5: Starting from the stop sign position, move the hand in a clockwise position, making several circles until the hand gets tired. Make the motion matter.

Step 6: Repeat the above steps with the opposite hand.

MOVEMENT INFORMATION

Movement Name
Hand Circles

Difficulty
Level 2
Where you'll see it

Physical therapy
Belly dance
Qigong

What it Wakes Up
Fingers, thumbs, wrists, palms
Forearms

Contraindications and Cautions
If you have carpal tunnel syndrome or other injuries of the hands or wrists, be particularly careful. Over-stretching can be dangerous.

Deepen the Movement
Perform this motion inside a bucket filled with rice.

In the Beginning...
Many beginners make this motion without fully lifting the hand. Be sure that on the hand's upward motion the fingers raise above the wrist as much as possible. Aim for a 90 degree angle between the back of the hand and the forearm.

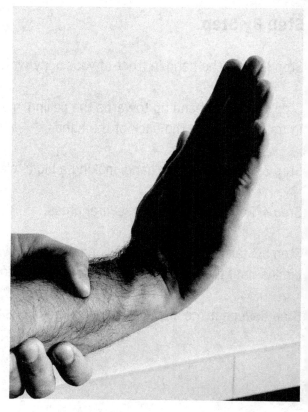

Additional Research
Search: "Belly Dancing Hand Circles"
Search: "Hand Circumduction"

28. FOREARM CIRCLES

Circumduct each forearm at the elbow.

After doing six strenuous exercises with the hands and fingers, it's time to rest the hands and bring your attention the elbow.

Circumducting the forearm at the elbow helps to distribute the synovial fluid of the elbow's ball and socket, lubricating and loosening this important joint. It also stretches the muscles of the upper arm including the bicep and tricep. It is great preparation for all forms of exercise and athletic activity.

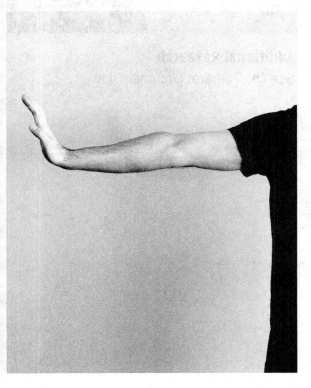

Step By Step

Step 1: Hold your arm out to the side, parallel to the floor.

Step 2: Keeping the elbow extended and the upper arm stable, circumduct the hand and forearm. Repeat the motion several times.

Step 3: Circumduct the forearm in the opposite direction several times.

Step 4: Switch arms and repeat the steps above.

MOVEMENT INFORMATION

Movement Name
Forearm Circles

Difficulty
Level 1

Where you'll see it
Warm up exercises
Indian Club exercises
Tennis
Physical therapy
Various types of dance
What it Wakes Up
Elbows
Biceps, triceps
Shoulders, deltoids

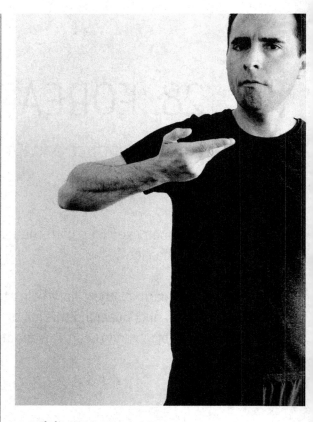

Contraindications and Cautions
If you have tennis elbow or any kind of elbow injury, talk to a doctor first.

Additional Research
Search: "Forearm Circumduction"

Deepen the Movement
Create a more complex movement by combining forearm circumduction with hand circumduction. There is a synergy to discover between the motion of the hand and that of the forearm.

In the Beginning...
Execute your full range of motion. Bring the forearm in very close to the chest on the way in and lock the elbow on the way out.

29. ARM CIRCLES

Circumduct each arm from the shoulder.

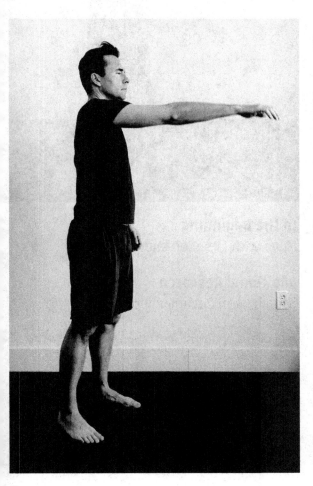

From the elbow, move up the arm to the shoulder joint, and make circles from there.

Step By Step

Step 1: Stand at Starting Position, feet shoulder width apart.

Step 2: Circumduct the entire arm in a backward direction. Bring the arm up behind your back, over the top of your head, and down in front of you, ending at the Starting Position.

Step 3: Repeat this motion several times, being sure to reach up through the shoulder, the bicep, and the side of the ribcage.

Step 4: Repeat the motion, moving in a forward direction, several times.

Step 5: Repeat the above steps using the opposite arm.

MOVEMENT INFORMATION

Movement Name
Arm Circles

Difficulty
Level 1

Where you'll see it
Swimming
Dance
Warmups
Physical therapy
Pilates
Martial arts

What it Wakes Up
Torso and abdomen
Upper back
Shoulder and shoulder girdle
Arms
Chest

Contraindications and Cautions
The shoulders are incredibly delicate. Be careful.

If you have any kind of shoulder injuries, see your doctor before doing this movement.

If you have any popping of joints, adjust the movement to avoid the popping sound.

Deepen the Movement
Practice the movement exploring different speeds, intensities, ranges of motion, etc.

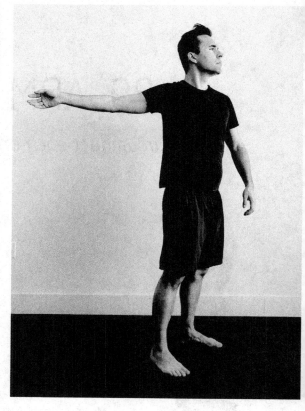

In the Beginning...
Move with intention and purpose.

Additional Research
Search: "Arm Circumduction"

30. STRAIGHTJACKETS

Hug yourself repeatedly in a straightjacket pose.

The Arm Circles can be physically demanding; it's now time to relax the arms and rest. The Straight-jacket appears at this point in the sequence to remove tension from the shoulders, arms, and back, thus giving your arms a rest before finishing the arm sequence at a higher intensity.

To get the full benefit of this movement, aim to create a slight slapping sound of the palm striking the torso.

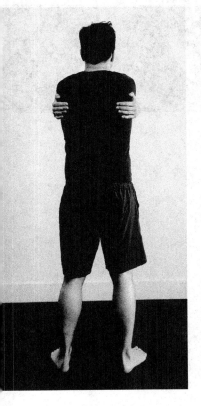

Step By Step

Step 1: Stand up straight and hold your arms out to the side like you're doing a Reverse Butterfly Press.

Step 2: Forcefully pull the arms forward, aligning the elbows over the top of one another, draping the arms across the sides and back. You will look like you've put on a straightjacket.

Step 3: You won't be able to hold the pose, since there's nothing to hold on to. Your arms will naturally start to fall back. Allow them to swing open to the Reverse Butterfly Pose again.

Step 4: Repeat the motion, this time switching which elbow is on top.

Step 5: Repeat the motion several times, switching the elbow each instance.

MOVEMENT INFORMATION

Movement Name
Straightjackets

Difficulty
Level 1

Where you'll see it
Cable crossovers
Yoga
What it Wakes Up
Back
Arms and elbows

Contraindications and Cautions
This is a generally safe movement.
If you have any shoulder or back injuries or chronic pain, talk to your doctor before executing this movement.

Deepen the Movement
Try to reach farther and/or slap the body harder each time.

In the Beginning...
If you can't get your arms around your body, either because of size or immobility, modify the movement according to your capability. Don't forget to switch which arm is on top.

Additional Research
None suggested.

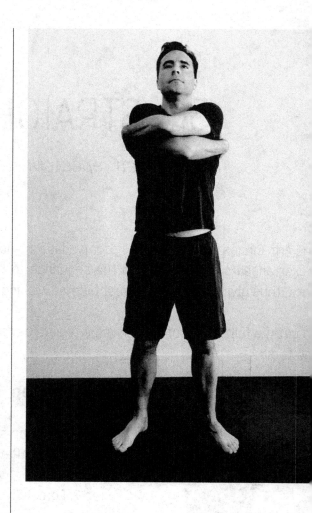

31. FRONT CRAWL STROKE

Circumduct the arms as if you're swimming in a forward crawl.

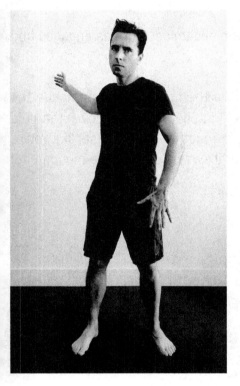

There was a short time in my life when I lived on a small island in the Caribbean, and every morning, at the start of the day, I would go for a swim in the ocean. It was one of the healthiest, happiest periods of my life. Swimming rejuvenated me, restored me, stimulated me, and strengthened me. Swimming is low impact on the joints, allows the body to move with a full range of motion, works the cardio/pulmonary system, and tones and strengthens the muscles.

Swimming may very well be the perfect form of physical activity.

Then one day my time in the Caribbean ended and it was back to New York City. There are no natural bodies of water to swim in, and public pools are not appealing for a host of reasons, chemicals being the main one. How could I create the experience of swimming while being in my studio apartment in Manhattan?

My answer was circumduction, the heart of the TheraQi method. Swimming is one of the few forms of exercise where circumduction plays the primary form of motion. Engaging in circumduction out-of-water recreates the experience of swimming somewhat and offers many of the same benefits. Doing the Front Crawl, the Backstroke, the Butterfly Stroke and the Reverse Butterfly Stroke while standing up tones the arms and abdominals, stimulates the cardio/pulmonary system, and increases overall range of motion.

Step By Step

Step 1: Stand in Starting Position, with feet shoulder width apart, arms down at the sides.

Step 2: Circumduct the right arm, back-to-front, by pulling the right arm up behind you and down in front. When you bring the arm down, move it forcefully as if you were performing a Karate-chop, or at a minimum pushing it through water.

Step 3: Circumduct the left arm, back-to-front, keeping the right arm where it is. Then switch back to the right arm. Alternate arms as if you're swimming.

Step 4: Repeat the forward stroke several times more. Keep the abdominal muscles engaged and move with intention.

Step 5: As the movement becomes more comfortable, speed up the movement and engage the shoulder girdle; move both arms at the same time (though still in opposition). Discover the fluid motion of the shoulder girdle as the arms move through space together. You will feel like you're swimming. Bring your attention to the hips and feel their natural sway. Continue the motion until you want to rest.

MOVEMENT INFORMATION

Movement Name
Front Crawl Stroke

Difficulty
Level 1

Where you'll see it
Swimming
What it Wakes Up
Arms
Chest
Back
Abdominals

Contraindications and Cautions
Extending the arm shifts the center of gravity of the body. The cantilevered arms can put pressure on the spine. Move slowly and intentionally at all times, keeping the head stable.
If you have any type of back or neck pain or injury, do not perform this movement without the supervision and permission of a doctor.
Move slowly. At no time should you feel any pain or discomfort.
Do not over-extend.
If you have any popping of the shoulder joint, adjust the movement to eliminate the popping.

Deepen the Movement
Practice the movement exploring different speeds, intensities, ranges of motion, etc.

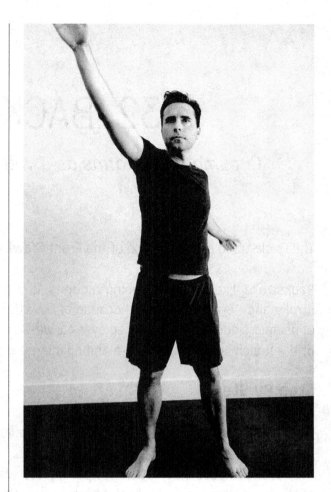

In the Beginning...
If you struggle with limited mobility, go easy on yourself. Move slowly with one arm at a time. As you build momentum, you can move both arms together simultaneously.

Additional Research
Search: "Front Crawl Stroke Swimming"

32. BACKSTROKE

Circumduct the arms as if you're swimming the backstroke.

The Backstroke is the reverse of the Front Crawl.

Backstroke, like other swimming motions, is a good fat-burner, but I particularly like the Backstroke and Reverse Butterfly because of how they open the shoulders and shoulder girdle. Many of us spend hours a day hunched over our desks or phones, and these reverse motions undo some of the hunch, improving posture and opening the chest.

Step By Step

Step 1: Stand in Starting Position, with feet shoulder width apart, arms down at the sides.

Step 2: Circumduct the right arm by pulling it forward and upward in front of the body; over the top of the head then down the back to return it to Starting Position. When you pull the arm up, move it forcefully, as if you were pulling on the cord to start a lawnmower.

Step 3: Repeat the backstroke with the left arm, keeping the right arm still.

Step 4: Repeat this backstroke several times. Move one arm and then the other. Keep the abdominal muscles engaged and move with intention.

Step 5: As the movement becomes more comfortable, speed up the movement and engage the shoulder girdle; move both arms at the same time (though still in opposition). Discover the fluid motion of the shoulder girdle as the arms move through space together. You will really feel like you're swimming. Bring your attention to the hips and feel their natural sway. Continue the motion until you want to rest.

MOVEMENT INFORMATION

Movement Name
Backstroke

Difficulty
Level 1

Where you'll see it
Swimming
What it Wakes Up
Arms
Chest
Back
Abdominals

Contraindications and Cautions
Extending the arm shifts the center of gravity of the body. The cantilevered arms can put pressure on the spine. Move slowly and intentionally at all times, keeping the head stable.
If you have any type of back or neck pain or injury, do not perform this movement without the supervision and permission of a doctor.
Move slowly. At no time should you feel any pain or discomfort.
Do not over-extend.
If you have any popping of the shoulder joint, adjust the movement to eliminate the popping.

Deepen the Movement
Practice the movement exploring different speeds, intensities, ranges of motion, etc.

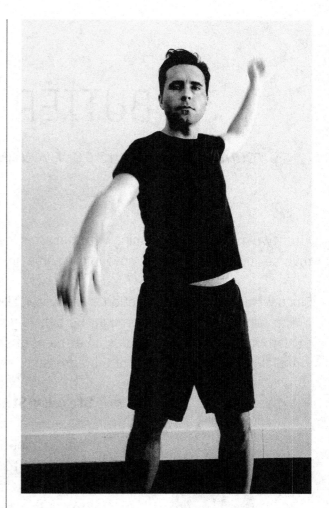

In the Beginning...
If you struggle with limited mobility, go easy on yourself. Move slowly with one arm at a time. As you build momentum, you can move both arms together simultaneously.

Additional Research
Search: "Backstroke Swimming"

33. BUTTERFLY STROKE

Circumduct the arms as if you're swimming the butterfly stroke.

After two motions of swimming with the arms in opposition, we have the Butterfly Stroke and its reverse, in which the arms move in the same direction at the same time.

Since we aren't doing this motion in the water, I like to modify it slightly by ending the motion with a clap. When the arms are brought up behind you and over your head, bring them down quickly to clap them together. This adds an element of shock to the motion, increasing the intensity and stimulating the bone density of the arms and hands.

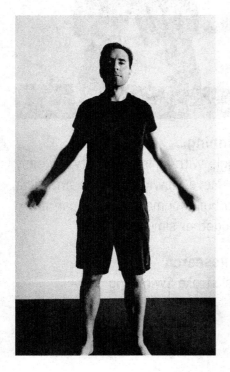

Step By Step

Step 1: Stand in Starting Position, feet shoulder width apart, arms down to the sides.

Step 2: In a single circular motion, pull the arms behind your body and pull them up overhead, before bringing them down with a loud clap in front of the body.

Step 3: Repeat this motion several times, clapping a few times at each of the Five Angles of Upper Body Fitness. Notice how when you change the location of the clap, it feels different in the arms and back. This means you're opening different parts of the back area and using different muscles in the back and chest.

Step 4: Repeat the motion until you get tired.

MOVEMENT INFORMATION

Movement Name
Butterfly Stroke

Difficulty
Level 2

Where you'll see it
Swimming
What it Wakes Up
Arms
Chest
Back
Abdominals

Contraindications and Cautions
Extending the arm shifts the center of gravity of the body. The cantilevered arms can put pressure on the spine. Move slowly and intentionally at all times, keeping the head stable.
If you have any type of back or neck pain or injury, do not perform this movement without the supervision and permission of a doctor.
Move slowly. At no time should you feel any pain or discomfort.
Do not over-extend.
If you have any popping of the shoulder joint, adjust the movement to eliminate the popping.

Deepen the Movement
Practice the movement exploring different speeds, intensities, ranges of motion, etc.

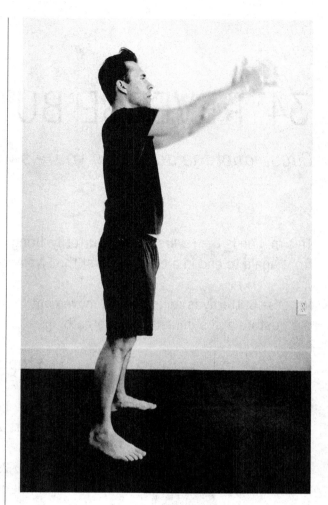

In the Beginning...
Do your best to make circles with the elbows, not just the wrists. The elbows need to get moving to really make this movement sing.

Additional Research
Search: "Butterfly Stroke Swimming"

34. REVERSE BUTTERFLY STROKE

Circumduct the arms as if you're swimming the reverse butterfly stroke

This motion is the reverse of the Butterfly. Bring the arms up the front, down the back and up the front again to end in a clap at one of the Five Angles of Upper Body Fitness.

Reverse Butterfly is an incredible movement to strengthen the shoulders and chest. It opens up the posture and stimulates your breathing.

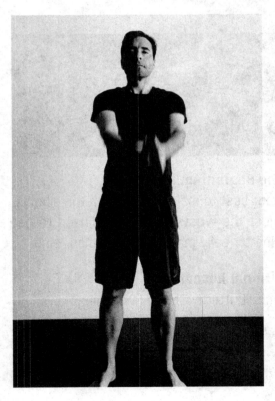

Step By Step

Step 1: Stand in Starting Position, feet shoulder width apart, arms down to the sides.

Step 2: In a single circular motion, pull the arms up in front of your body and overhead, down behind you, and up again before ending with a loud clap.

Step 3: Repeat this motion several times, clapping a few times in each of the Five Angles of Upper Body Fitness.

Step 4: Repeat the motion until you get tired.

MOVEMENT INFORMATION

Movement Name
Reverse Butterfly Stroke

Difficulty
Level 2

Where you'll see it
Swimming
What it Wakes Up
Arms
Chest
Back
Abdominals

Contraindications and Cautions
Extending the arm shifts the center of gravity of the body. The cantilevered arms can put pressure on the spine. Move slowly and intentionally at all times, keeping the head stable.
If you have any type of back or neck pain or injury, do not perform this movement without the supervision and permission of a doctor. Move slowly. At no time should you feel any pain or discomfort.
Do not over-extend.
If you have any popping of the shoulder joint, adjust the movement to eliminate the popping.

Deepen the Movement
Practice the movement exploring different speeds, intensities, ranges of motion, etc.

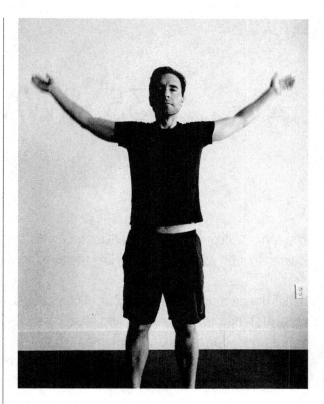

In the Beginning...
Do your best to make circles with the elbows, not just the wrists. The elbows need to get moving to make this movement sing.

Additional Research
Search: "Reverse Butterfly Stroke Swimming"

35. SWAN ARMS

Flap your arms up and down over your head.

The arms section of the sequence ends with a movement called Swan Arms. This deceptively easy looking motion will have you "feeling the burn" in your deltoid muscles before you can say "Swan Lake."

Ballet dancers and ballet workout aficionados swear by Swan Arms as one of the best movements to stretch and tone the arms and shoulders. Just because this movement supports graceful, elongated arms, don't think for a moment that it's easy. Swan Arms is a very intense movement that activates the shoulder muscles, making it a great warmup for handstands, pull-ups, and various upper body exercises.

Don't be too worried about form. My Swan Arms look more like Frog Legs, but the activation and benefits are the same.

Step By Step

Step 1: Stand in Starting Position, feet shoulder width apart, arms to the sides.

Step 2: Raise the elbows out to the sides, placing the upper arms at 90 degree angles to the torso, parallel to the floor, palms facing outward. Keep the hands and lower part of the arms extended but loose.

Step 3: Repeatedly raise the elbows up towards the ears, raising the arms up overhead to bring the backs of the hands together; then lower the elbows back to shoulder height. Don't let the elbows drop below the shoulders when the arms come back down.

Step 4: Repeat this up-and-down motion several times until your arms get too tired to continue.

MOVEMENT INFORMATION

Movement Name
Swan Arms

Difficulty
Level 3

Where you'll see it
Ballet
What it Wakes Up
Arms
Chest
Back
Abdominals
Shoulders

Contraindications and Cautions
If you have any type of back or shoulder
pain or injury, do not perform this movement
without the supervision and permission of a
doctor.
At no time should you feel any pain or discomfort.
Do not over-extend.
If you have any popping of the shoulder joint,
adjust the movement to eliminate the popping.

Deepen the Movement
Practice the movement exploring different
speeds, intensities, ranges of motion, etc.

In the Beginning...
Use a mirror to check your form.

Additional Research
Search: "Ballet Swan Arms Exercise"

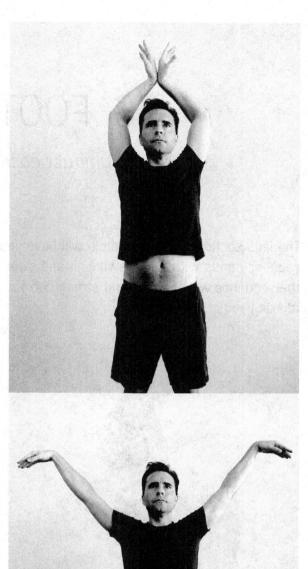

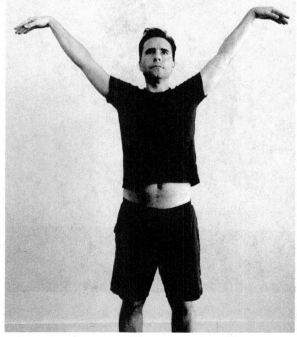

36. FOOT CIRCLES

Circumduct each foot at the ankle.

The legs section of the sequence will have you circumduct the feet, lower legs, and thighs. The sequence ends with a few swinging and sweeping motions of the legs and feet. This section of the sequence will energize and strengthen your lower body, increasing your range of motion and relaxing you at the same time.

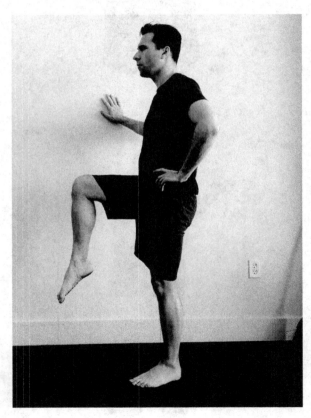

Foot circumduction is similar to hand circumduction: make as big of a circle as you can, and feel the stretch all the way through. Do your best to push the foot down and pull it up as you go through the complete 360 degree motion.

To get the full benefit of this motion, I highly recommend performing the movement barefoot. This will give you the most freedom of movement to experience each of the ten toes in their individual ranges of motion. You'll even see the toes begin to make very subtle wave motions, like the fingers did in the Finger Wave. It wakes up the brain to discover the complex biomechanics of the feet. Just like the hands, our feet are miracles that we take for granted. Foot Circles give our feet the love they deserve.

Step By Step

Step 1: From either a standing or seated position, raise one leg and point the toes of that foot down into the ground. If you require support when standing on one leg, feel free to use a chair or lean against the wall.

Step 2: Circumduct the foot in a wide circle, tracing a cone-like shape through space. Repeat this motion several times, stretching the feet and toes as you go.

Step 3: Repeat the circumduction moving in the opposite direction.

Step 4: Repeat the above steps with the opposite foot.

MOVEMENT INFORMATION

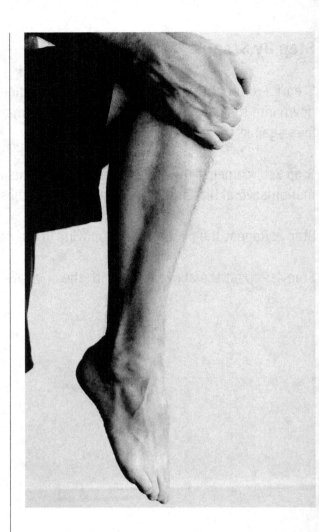

Movement Name
Foot Circles

Difficulty
Level 1

Where you'll see it
Physical therapy
Dance
What it Wakes Up
Toes, feet
Calves
Shins

Contraindications and Cautions
As with all movements, go carefully. Push yourself but don't overdo it. I have occasionally gone overboard with this movement and ended up with cramps in my toes or calf.

Deepen the Movement
Do your best to exaggerate the individuality of each toe.
Discover how each toe is distinct and try to create space between the toes as you perform the movement.

In the Beginning...
If you struggle with the movement, find a circle to trace about a foot in diameter.

Additional Research
Search: "Foot Circumduction"

37. LOWER LEG CIRCLES

Circumduct each lower leg at the knee.

his is a simple, but enjoyable, movement that lubricates and opens the knee. When performed tanding on one leg, it's a great exercise for learning balance and strengthening the opposite leg.

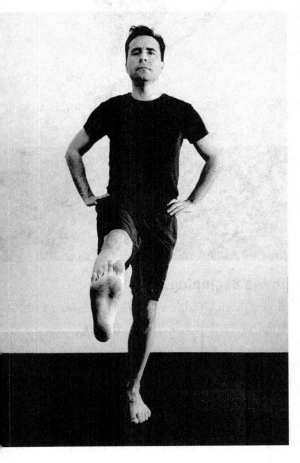

Step By Step

Step 1: Stand on one leg, with the lifted knee slightly higher than the waist. Hold the raised knee for support and balance if you prefer.

Step 2: Circumduct the lower part of the raised leg in as wide a circle as you can. Aim to straighten the leg entirely when the leg is extended, and pull the foot as close as possible to the body on the return. Repeat the motion several times.

Step 3: Reverse the direction of the circumduction. Repeat this motion several times.

Step 4: Switch legs and repeat the above steps.

MOVEMENT INFORMATION

Movement Name
Lower Leg Circles

Difficulty
Level 2

Where you'll see it
Qigong
Pilates
Ballet and dance
What it Wakes Up
Calves
Knees
Feet
Thighs
Hamstrings

Contraindications and Cautions
This is a generally safe movement.
Go slow and end the movement if you encounter any pain.
If you have any knee injuries or chronic pain, talk to your doctor before executing this movement.

Deepen the Movement
The key here is to extend the full range of motion.
Notice that when you extend the leg outward your thigh will want to drop. Intensify the movement by intentionally raising the thigh as you extend the lower leg on the outward part of the circle.

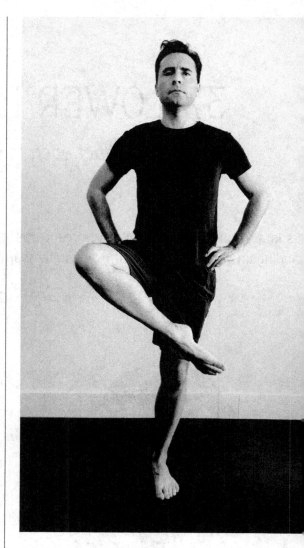

In the Beginning...
If you have trouble with your balance, execut the movement while lying down.

Additional Research
None suggested.

38. FRONT-FACING LEG CIRCLES

Circumduct each leg in front of your body.

This movement is a challenging one. Given how much the leg weighs, the circumduction of the entire leg requires the use of all the muscles in the lower body, making it an excellent fat-burner and cardio-pulmonary enhancer. This one works the muscles of the thigh and repeated use will give you shapely, muscular legs.

Unless you have the flexibility of a ninja, you won't be able to extend your leg fully, but it's something to aspire towards. Most people will need to bend the knee, circumducting the thigh bone while the lower leg hangs loose from the knee. As you gain strength, try extending the lower leg as much possible.

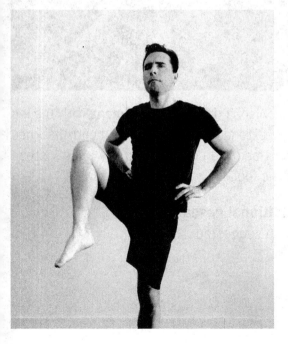

Step By Step

Step 1: Stand in Starting Position with one leg extended in front of you. The straighter the leg extension, the more challenging the movement.

Step 2: Using the extended foot as a guide, circumduct the extended leg. Repeat the motion several times.

Step 3: Circumduct the leg several times more, moving in the opposite direction.

Step 4: Repeat the above steps with the opposite leg.

MOVEMENT INFORMATION

Movement Name
Front Leg Circles

Difficulty
Level 3

Where you'll see it
Ballet
Dance
Martial arts
Qigong
Physical therapy
Pilates

What it Wakes Up
All the muscles and joints of the lower body.

Contraindications and Cautions
This is a generally safe movement.
Go slow and end the movement if you encounter any pain.
If you have any knee injuries or chronic pain, talk to your doctor before executing this movement.
If you have any popping of joints, adjust the movement to avoid the popping sound.

Deepen the Movement
Practice the movement exploring different speeds, intensities, ranges of motion, etc.

In the Beginning…
You may perform this movement lying down on the back until you get the hang of the mo-

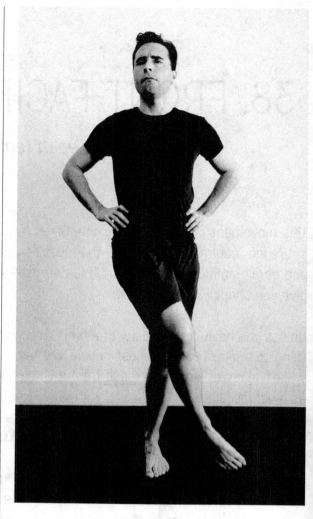

tion. Also, if doing the movement with the leg fully extended is too difficult, bend the knee and trace the circles using the knee instead of the foot.

Additional Research
None suggested.

39. REAR-FACING LEG CIRCLES

Circumduct each leg behind your body.

This motion is the reverse of the last motion. It provides a very intense workout for the butt, hamstrings, and lower back. When performed without support standing on one leg, it's also a great movement to improve balance.

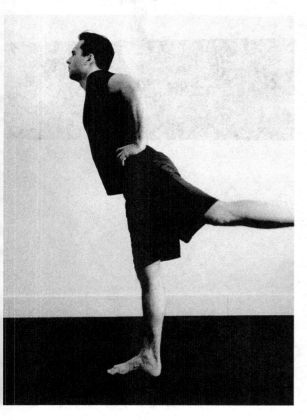

Step By Step

Step 1: Stand in Starting Position with one leg extended behind the body.

Step 2: Using the extended foot as a guide, circumduct the extended leg. Repeat the motion several times.

Step 3: Circumduct the leg several times more, moving in the opposite direction.

Step 4: Repeat the above steps with the opposite leg.

MOVEMENT INFORMATION

Movement Name
Rear-facing Leg Circles

Difficulty
Level 3

Where you'll see it
Ballet
Pilates
Dance

What it Wakes Up
All the muscles and joints of the lower body.

Contraindications and Cautions
This is a generally safe movement.
Go slow and end the movement if you encounter any pain.
If you have any knee injuries or chronic pain, talk to your doctor before executing this movement.
If you have any popping of joints, adjust the movement to avoid the popping sound.

Deepen the Movement
Practice the movement exploring different speeds, intensities, ranges of motion, etc.

In the Beginning...
If you have trouble keeping your balance, hold on to a railing or the back of a chair for support.

Additional Research
Search: "Standing Leg Circles for Hip Mobility"

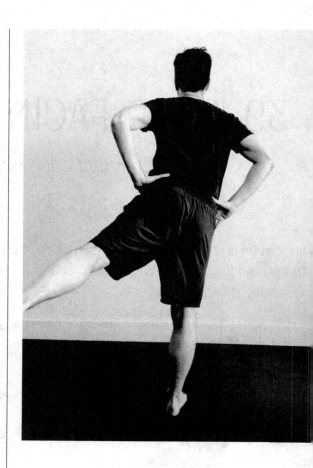

40. STANDING LEG CURLS

Kick each foot up to your butt.

This is one of the easiest movements in the sequence and a great way to loosen, lubricate, and stretch the knee. This move can be done as a simple up/down flex/extend or as a circumduction.

Step By Step

One leg at a time:

Step 1: In one smooth motion, kick the right leg up behind you and lower it back down, boot-to-butt. Repeat several times.

Step 2: Repeat the motion with the opposite leg.

Alternating legs:

Step 1: Stand at Starting Position, feet shoulder width apart.

Step 2: Shift your weight onto the left foot, and kick the right foot up behind you, boot-to-butt, before returning it to the floor.

Step 3: As you place the right foot back on the floor, shift your weight to the right foot, and then lift the left foot up boot-to-butt before bringing it back down.

Step 4: Repeat the motion several times shifting weight from one foot to the other and kicking the opposite leg up behind you. Be sure to keep the knees pointing down to the ground. Don't let the thigh come up behind you.

MOVEMENT INFORMATION

Movement Name
Standing Leg Curls

Difficulty
Level 1

Where you'll see it
Yoga
Dance
Weightlifting
What it Wakes Up
Knees
Hamstrings
Calves
Butt

Contraindications and Cautions
This is a generally safe movement.
If you have any knee injuries or chronic pain, talk to your doctor before executing this movement.

Deepen the Movement
Move to yoga "Butterfly Pose" or "Kneeling Pose".

In the Beginning...
Hold on to the back of a chair for balance if necessary.

Additional Research
Search: "Standing Leg Curls"

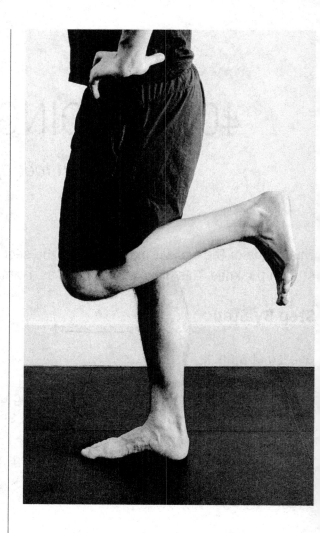

41. LEG SWINGS

Swing each leg back and forth.

Much like the standing leg curls, this movement is simple to execute. Simply swing your leg back and forth while standing on the other leg. That doesn't make it effortless, however. The leg has considerable weight, almost 15% of your total body, and engaging this movement vigorously can raise the heart rate considerably. It's an excellent movement to tone the butt and thighs while releasing tension and stretching the hamstring and thigh. This movement is also an excellent way to develop a sense of balance and stability.

Step By Step

Step 1: Stand up straight with your weight on one leg and the other leg slightly lifted off the floor.

Step 2: Swing the lifted leg back and forth. Aim to lift the leg as high as possible at both ends of the swing. Throughout the movement, pull back the toes to point them at the knee, stretching through the foot, which will in turn create a stretch through the hamstring as you swing.

Step 3: Repeat this motion several times, adjusting the speed, intensity, range of motion, and other fitness factors.

Step 4: Switch legs and repeat all of the above.

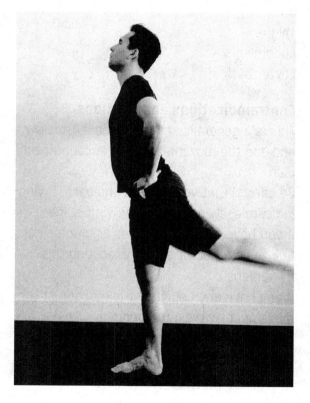

MOVEMENT INFORMATION

Movement Name
Leg Swings

Difficulty
Level 2
Where you'll see it
Gymnastics
Aerobics
Pilates
Physical therapy
Martial arts
Dance
What it Wakes Up
Hamstrings
Butt
Thighs
Abdominals
Lower back

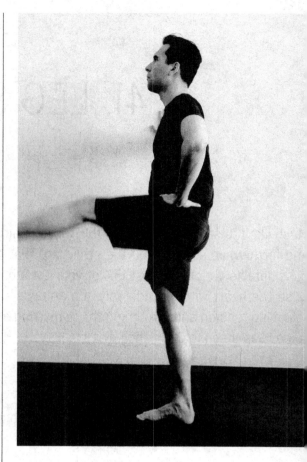

Contraindications and Cautions
This is a generally safe movement. Go slow and end the movement if you encounter any pain.
Be careful that you support the back. Swinging carelessly could damage your spine.
If you have any knee injuries or chronic pain, talk to your doctor before executing this movement.
If you have any popping of joints, adjust the movement to avoid the popping sound.

Deepen the Movement
Kick as high as you can in both directions, keeping the leg as straight as possible.
For a deeper movement, research the "Front Scale" and "Rear Scale" in gymnastics.

In the Beginning...
Hold on to a railing or the back of a chair for balance.

Additional Research
Search: "Leg Swings"
Search: "Front Scale Back Scale Gymnastics"

42. STANDING DONKEY KICKS

Kick each leg behind your body as if you're an angry donkey.

Standing Donkey Kicks are very similar to the Leg Swings we learned in the last lesson. Donkey Kicks are simply Leg Swings performed with the knee bent to 90 degrees.

Donkey Kicks are a powerful butt building exercise if done intensely and for a long set of repetitions. That doesn't mean you have to go crazy. Doing them gently opens up the hip and hamstring making it like a stretch.

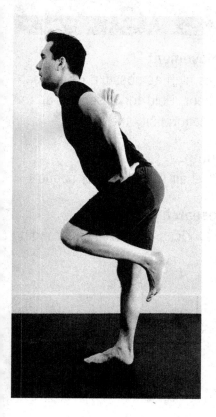

Step By Step

Step 1: Stand up straight with your weight on one leg and the other leg slightly lifted off the floor.

Step 2: Lean forward, and raise the lower part of the lifted leg to 90 degrees. Then thrust the lifted leg back and forth, keeping the knee at a right angle. Aim to lift the leg as high as possible at both ends of the swing. On the way forward, focus on bringing the knee as high up as possible. On the way back lift the heel up towards the ceiling. Throughout the movement, pull back the toes to point them at the knee, stretching through the foot. This will in turn create a stretch through the hamstring as you swing.

Step 3: Repeat this motion several times, adjusting the speed, intensity, range of motion, and other fitness factors.

Step 4: Switch legs and repeat the steps above.

MOVEMENT INFORMATION

Movement Name
Standing Donkey Kicks
Difficulty
Level 2

Where you'll see it
Gymnastics
Aerobics
Pilates
Physical therapy
Martial arts
Ballet
Jazz dance
Weightlifting/Bodybuilding

What it Wakes Up
Hamstrings
Butt
Thighs
Abdominals
Lower back

Contraindications and Cautions
This is a generally safe movement. Go slow and end the movement if you encounter any pain.
Be careful that you support the back. Swinging carelessly could damage your spine.
If you have any knee injuries or chronic pain, talk to your doctor before executing this movement.
If you have any popping of joints, adjust the movement to avoid the popping sound.

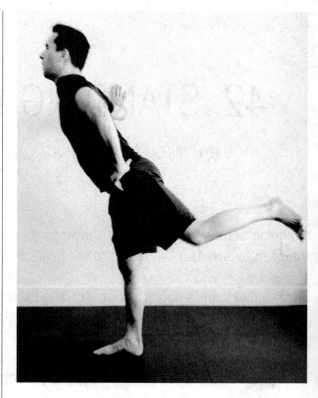

Deepen the Movement
Raise the leg as high as possible while keeping the knee bent. Hold for a second at the rear extension to intensify the squeeze.

In the Beginning...
Lean on a wall, chair or counter for support.

Additional Research
Search: "Donkey Kicks Exercise" or "Standing Donkey Kicks"

43. PAW BACK

Sweep each foot on the ground from front to back,
as if you're kicking up sand behind you.

This last movement, which fully and finally activates the butt and legs, is a silly, awkward, and slightly embarrassing movement. This movement basically imitates the movement a dog or cat makes when covering its poo. Despite the silliness, it's a powerful movement to tone the legs and butt, and when done for a long time will elevate the heart rate.

This movement only works on carpet or hardwood floors while wearing socks or toe-shoes. You could do it at the beach in the sand, but if you do it in grass or gravel you'll make a mess. It's also one of the movements I would not want to do barefoot, as it would probably burn your skin from the friction. Doing it in shoes may be difficult due to too much friction.

Step By Step

Step 1: Stand up straight with your weight on one leg and the other leg slightly lifted off the floor.

Step 2: In one smooth motion, swing the lifted leg forward (like in a leg swing) keeping the toes pointed up, then bring the leg down and back, sweeping the foot across the floor; press into the floor as you drag the leg behind you. As you get to the natural point where your foot lifts up, bring the leg up and repeat.

Step 3: Repeat this motion several times, adjusting the speed, intensity, range of motion, and other fitness factors.

Step 4: Switch legs and repeat all steps above.

MOVEMENT INFORMATION

Movement Name
Paw Back

Difficulty
Level 2

Where you'll see it
The local dog run.
Runners use this as a training exercise.

What it Wakes Up
The entire lower body.

Contraindications and Cautions
This is a generally safe movement.
Go slow and end the movement if you encounter any pain.
Be careful that you support the back. Swinging carelessly could damage your spine.
If you have any knee injuries or chronic pain, talk to your doctor before executing this movement.
If you have any popping of joints, adjust the movement to avoid the popping sound.

Deepen the Movement
The harder you press into the floor the more intense the movement will be.

In the Beginning...
Don't worry about getting the motion exactly right. Focus on dragging the foot backwards to create tension and resistance in the hamstring and butt.

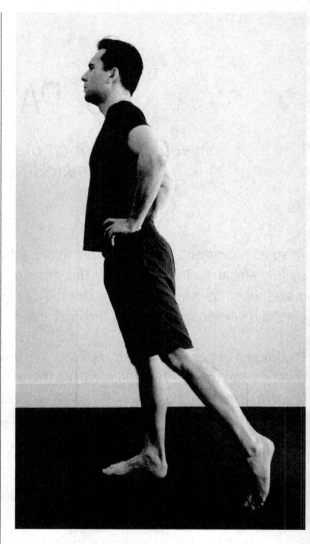

Additional Research
Search: "Paw Back Running Exercise"

44. LION FACE

Make a face as if you're a lion.

Lion Face is a modified set of yoga motions which stretch and strengthen the face muscles, including the jaw and tongue. There are over 42 muscles in the face, and this movement awakens all of them. I love doing this movement in the mornings or any time I need to release tension in the jaw, cheeks, and forehead.

Raise your eyebrows up and down to understand how your eyebrows are connected to your scalp. Wiggle your scalp and ears. Now open your eyes wide and tighten up your cheeks. Scrunch your eyes like you're squinting.

Open your mouth as wide as you can, and move the muscles in your cheeks and around your lips. Pucker your lips like you're smoking. Now open your mouth and stick out your tongue as far as you can. When your eyes are wide, your mouth is opened, and your tongue is out, you will look like a real lion.

The Jaw

Pull your tongue back in your mouth, but keeping your mouth open wide, start to explore the movement of your jaw. The obvious movement of the jaw is up and down like you're chewing, but there are other ways of moving your jaw to explore.

First, with your mouth slightly open and your teeth only slightly parted, push your jaw forward so your bottom teeth stick out past your top teeth. Jutting it out as far as possible, tighten the muscles in your neck at the same time and pucker your lips. Now pull your jaw back in towards the back of your throat. Do this a couple of times, sliding forward and back like the drawer of a cabinet.

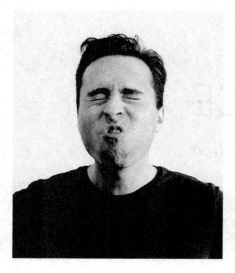

Then, try shifting your jaw from side to side, as far right as possible, then as far left as possible.

Spend some time playing around with your face and jaw to explore the different ways your face can move. Try tightening, stretching, scrunching, and wiggling. Open and close your mouth and eyes, and stick out your tongue several times. Just enjoy the stretching of your face; feel the tension leaving your face and scalp as you do this movement. Your jaw should be relaxing. This is a great exercise for people who clench their jaw when they sleep or who suffer from other tight-jaw symptoms.

Step By Step

Step 1: Open the mouth and eyes as wide as you can.

Step 2: Keeping everything wide and open, tighten the face muscles around the eyes, mouth, cheek and neck.

Step 3: Stick out the tongue as far as you can. Flick it in and out a few times for good measure.

Step 4: Relax the face and now raise and lower the eyebrows a few times.

Step 5: Scrunch the face up as tight as you can.

Step 6: Now move everything around all at once, letting the face go crazy with movement. Wiggle the jaw up and down, forward and back, side to side.

Step 7: Take a deep breath and relax. Feel the aliveness in your face: the decrease of tension and the increase of circulation and energy.

MOVEMENT INFORMATION

Movement Name
Lion Face

Difficulty
Level 1

Where you'll see it
Yoga
Face Yoga

What it Wakes Up
Face
Eyes
Jaw

Contraindications and Cautions
Be gentle with the eyes. You can hurt yourself if you are not careful.
Adjust the movement of the jaw to avoid any popping.

Deepen the Movement
Do not deepen this movement. Perform only what is comfortable.

In the Beginning...
Learn to use the feeling in the face to guide the movement, rather than trying to do it a certain way. Then, go to the mirror to see what you've been doing.

Additional Research
Search: "Face Yoga" or "Lion's Breath Pose"

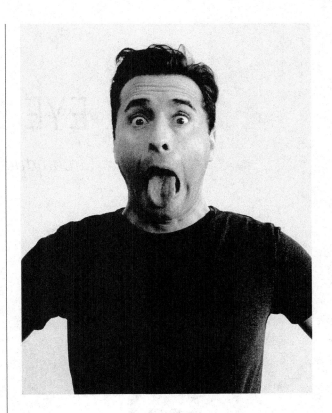

45. EYE CIRCLES

Circumduct the eyes.

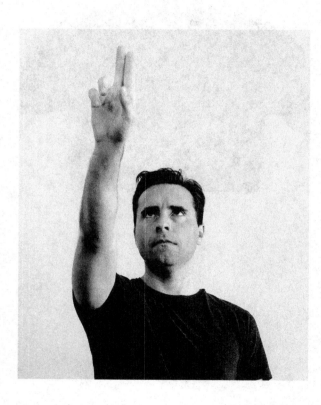

Most of the time in modern life we are staring straight ahead. We stare at books, we stare at screens, we stare at the highway when we drive. Yet the eyes are designed with a very wide range of motion, and there's something magical about waking up the potential movement of the eyes.

Like the rest of the sequence, we use circumduction whenever possible to wake up the body and mind. The eyes are attached at one end and free on the other, and are thus able to circumduct. The only challenge with circumducting the eyes is that because they are so short, the cone shape is hard to visualize. Imagine the cone shape extending beyond the eyes. We make that visualization easier by using the hands as a guide.

The hands are also used as a guide for safety reasons. Free style eye circles can easily over extend, potentially causing strain or injury. Extending and circumducting the arm in front of the face helps keep the movement controlled and intentional.

I find this movement releases a lot of subtle tension in my face and head. In my experience, Eye Circles improve my mood, clear my mind, and prevent headaches. They make an excellent mid-day break activity.

Step By Step

Step 1: Stand up in Starting Position. Extend one arm out in front of you, palm facing forward with two fingers raised.

Step 2: Slowly circumduct the extended arm, keeping the eyes fixated on the two raised fingers.

Step 3: Expand the circumference of the arm circumduction until the circles are very wide and the eye is experiencing its full range of motion.

Step 4: Come back to the center and start the ever-widening circles again, this time moving in the opposite direction.

Step 5: End by bringing the fingers up to the nose and back out, in order to provide a "cross-eye" stretch.

MOVEMENT INFORMATION

Movement Name
Eye Circles

Difficulty
Level 1

Where you'll see it
Eye yoga

What it Wakes Up
Eyes, face, head

Contraindications and Cautions
Move cautiously and intentionally. The eye is incredibly delicate and especially in the beginning you want to be gentle. Building up tolerance and strength in the eye is essential. Don't push yourself with this one.

Deepen the Movement
Do not deepen this movement.

In the Beginning...
Always follow the hand.

Additional Research
Search: "Eye Yoga"

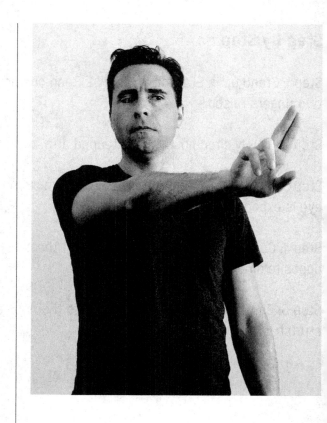

46. HULA SQUAT

Squat and hula at the same time.

Until now, the sequence has mostly focused on isolation movements. To maximize your muscle building and fat burning potential, it's important to know how to perform a selection of compound exercises. Compound exercises are movements that use the entire body. They tend to be more physically demanding than isolations.

There are some major benefits to compounds, beyond just the calorie-burning and muscle-building aspects. Compounds strengthen your core, which means they work your middle. Compounds also make you better at your daily activities, like lifting groceries and doing other chores, because they require the exertion of the entire body. Many forms of strength training and athletics depend upon compound movements. They aren't the focus of the TheraQi method, because they can be studied in detail in many other places. The problem with compounds is that they are physically demanding the average person isn't prepared to do them. TheraQi provides a foundation for compound movements that's largely missing in the general fitness conversation.

There is a type of bodyweight exercise called an "Air Squat." In the Air Squat, you squat to where your hips are just slightly below your knees, and then you come back up. This is a very popular bodyweight exercise that you'll see performed by trainers.

When working out at home, however, I'm not a fan of the traditional Air Squat. I feel like Air Squats are stuck in the flex/extend paradigm of traditional fitness. You squat down, you come back up. Flex, extend. I personally find it boring, and I also find that it puts a lot of pressure on my joints. I wanted to find a way to experience the benefits of squats that was more comfortable, easy, and fun, and that took advantage of the range of motion developed elsewhere in the sequence.

Enter the Hula Squat.

The Hula Squat is a compound exercise that blends the motion of Hip Hula with a squat. Remember that a squat means you bend at the waist and you bend at the knees. In this movement, as you swing your hips behind you, stick out your arms and squat at the same time, coming back up as you swing your hips to the front again.

Some Hula hooping athletes have a different version of the Hula Squat in which they squat while doing a Pelvis Hula. The TheraQi version of the Hula Squat is more accurately a modified Air Squat in which the hips move in a large circle. It is very different from the Hula Squat you might find elsewhere.

The Hip Hula Squat gets the heart rate going, and if done for a long enough time, will really burn some calories.

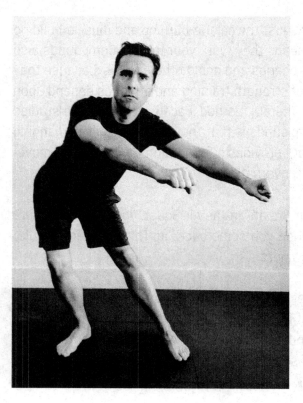

Step By Step

Step 1: Move yourself in a Hip Hula several times to get some momentum going.

Step 2: As you swing your hips behind you, bend your knees and waist to drop the pelvis, as if you were trying to sit down.

Step 3: Keep the momentum of the Hula going, and as your hips swing to the front, straighten the knees and hips to return to a standing position.

Step 4: Repeat the motion several times. Don't go any deeper than you feel comfortable.

Step 5: Repeat the motion several times, moving in the other direction.

MOVEMENT INFORMATION

Movement Name
Hip Hula Squats

Difficulty
Level 4

Where you'll see it
Jazz
Dance
Hula hooping
What it Wakes Up
Abdominals
Lower body

Contraindications and Cautions
Compound exercises are more intense than the other movements in this sequence. Be sure you have cleared with your doctor that you're ready for advanced levels of exercise and exertion.
If performed carelessly, this movement can be hard on the knees.

Deepen the Movement
Research and advance into Hindu Squats or Air Squats.

In the Beginning...
Go slow and move carefully until you are comfortable with the motion.

Additional Research
None suggested.

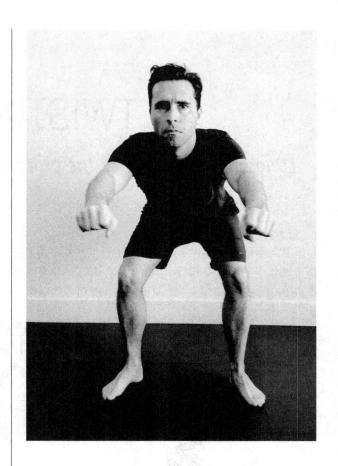

47. TWISTING LUNGE

Lunge from one side to the other while doing an upper torso twist.

Lunges are a staple of many physical fitness programs. A lunge refers to any movement where one leg is pointed forward with a bent knee and a flat foot, and the other leg is behind the body pointing backward, with the foot up on the toes and the heel up to the ceiling.

In this version of a lunge we add a Torso Twist, which puts less stress on your knees and makes the movement more comfortable, though admittedly, it requires more coordination. This twisting lunge is an excellent advanced move to improve balance and coordination while increasing muscle and burning calories.

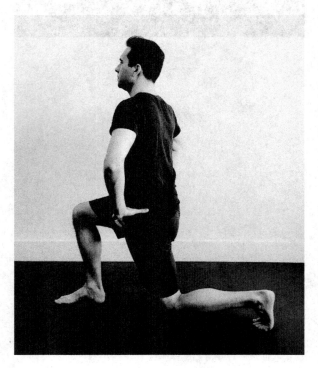

Step By Step

Step 1: Stand with the feet very wide apart.

Step 2: Gently perform a very loose, easy Torso Twist with the legs spread very wide.

Step 3: As you twist to the right side, turn the entire torso to the right, pivoting your feet to the right as well, and as you turn, bend the knees and drop the pelvis into a lunge. Be sure to keep the knee fully behind the ankle. You may struggle to keep your balance. Use a chair for support if required. Finish the Torso Twist at the bottom of the movement.

Step 4: Continue the Torso Twist by unwinding the torso and starting to twist back in the opposite direction. Raise yourself up as you do, so that you're fully raised again as your arms are at the midpoint of the twist. You're now preparing to go down the other side.

Step 5: Continue the Torso Twist to the left, and continue the steps above to twist and lunge together.

Step 6: Repeat the motion until you get tired.

MOVEMENT INFORMATION

Movement Name
Twisting Lunge

Difficulty
Level 4

Where you'll see it
Physical training
Gymnastics
Yoga
What it Wakes Up
The entire body.

Contraindications and Cautions
Compound exercises are more intense than the other movements in this sequence. Be sure you have cleared with your doctor that you're ready for advanced levels of exercise and exertion.

If not performed carefully this can be a dangerous movement, causing damage to the neck, spine and knees. Move slowly and intentionally at all times, keeping the head stable.

If you have any type of neck pain or injury, do not perform this movement without the supervision and permission of a doctor.

Move slowly. At no time should you feel any pain or discomfort.

Do not over extend the knee beyond the ankle.

Deepen the Movement
Focus on form and intentionality.

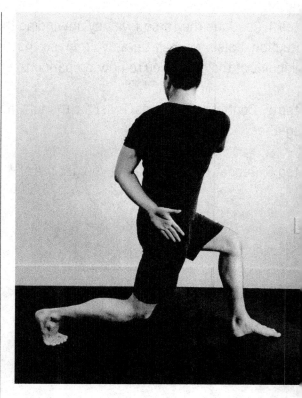

In the Beginning...
Use a mirror to check your form.
Use any type of support you need to get into and out of the movement.
Be very careful with the back.

Additional Research
Search: "Twisting Lunges"

48. SIT & RISE

Sit cross-legged and rise off the floor.

Sit & Rise improves your ability to sit and rise from the floor with as little support as necessary. For someone very fit, it's easy to lift oneself from a cross-legged position using only the feet. Less fit people may require the use of a knee, hand, or elbow. By practicing this movement, you can get a good sense of how fit you are.

It's also a test of how long you're likely to live.

In 2014, a group of Brazilian doctors published research in the European Journal of Cardiovascular Prevention that linked performance on this movement with mortality. The less support the patient needed to lift themselves up, the longer that person was expected to live.

The doctors were quoted as saying about the study:

"It is well known that aerobic fitness is strongly related to survival, but our study also shows that maintaining high levels of body flexibility, muscle strength, power-to-body weight ratio and co-ordination are not only good for performing daily activities but have a favorable influence on life expectancy."

The Sit & Rise is a powerful exercise not only for diagnosing your current health, but for keeping your lower body strong, flexible, and stable.

Step By Step

Step 1: Sit down on the floor in a cross-legged style.

Step 2: Get up off the floor and stand up, twisting yourself upwards. Ideally, you would do this without using any part of your body except your feet. Shift your weight to the feet; push down into the floor with your feet; push up the body and start to "unwind" from the cross-legged position; by the time your legs are fully extended you will be facing the wall behind you from when you were sitting down. If you need to use your arms, legs, or a chair to help yourself up, go ahead.

Step 3: Continue twisting as you lower your body into the cross-legged position once again. You'll be facing the original direction.

Step 4: Repeat until you get tired.

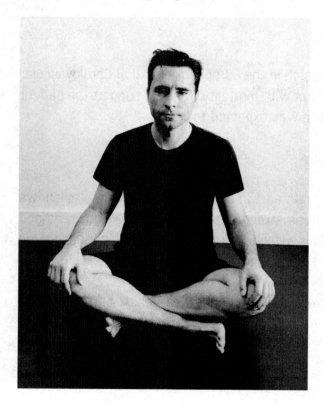

MOVEMENT INFORMATION

Movement Name
Sit & Rise

Difficulty
Level 4

Where you'll see it
Physical therapy
Martial arts
What it Wakes Up
The entire lower body

Contraindications and Cautions
Compound exercises are more intense than the other movements in this sequence. Be sure you have cleared with your doctor that you're ready for advanced levels of exercise and exertion.
This exercise can be very hard on the feet, knees, and ankles if you're not prepared for it. Move carefully. Under no circumstances should you support all your weight on your knees/ankles until you are ready.

Deepen the Movement
Practice the movement until you can easily "pop" up and down repeatedly in one smooth motion, without resting your butt on the ground.

In the Beginning...
Use whatever props or support you need to get yourself up off the floor. The point is to get up and go back down.

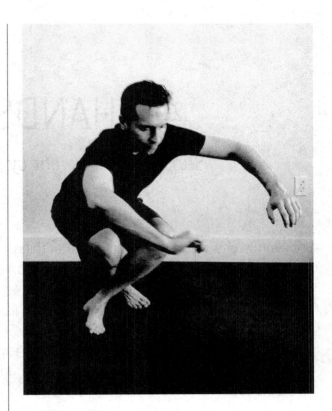

Additional Research
Search: "Sit and Rise Test"

49. HANDSTANDING

Support your weight by pressing into the floor.

Standing is one of the most fundamental things our bodies do. It's one of those things we just take for granted, forgetting that standing is a very physically demanding activity that requires immense strength, coordination, and balance. As toddlers, we learn to stand before we learn to perform more complex lower body movements like walking or running.

It's such a mystery to me that while we don't expect a child to run before she can stand, we do expect adults to be able to perform all kinds of upper body exercises without being able to stand on the hands.

If you lack the strength, coordination, balance, stamina, and other fitness factors to stand in place with your hands and arms, why on earth would you think it's a good idea to perform more complex tasks? This is the upper body equivalent of trying to run before you can walk.

Handstanding is the foundation of upper body strength. If you want a strong upper body, hand-standing is all there is to do. Practice daily for twenty minutes. You'll have a fantastic upper body in twelve weeks and every other upper body exercise will become effortless. Seriously, if you can't handstand, don't bother with anything else.

I use the word handstanding intentionally. If I say "Do a handstand" you have a very specific image of someone completely upside down, with their legs in the air and their body perfectly straight. Well that's fine and good, but just like a baby doesn't just wake up one day and stand on her two feet, you'll not be doing a perfect handstand anytime soon. It takes time to overcome a lifetime of upper body atrophy. That said, barring a disability or other medical condition, you are more than capable of handstanding: supporting your bodyweight with yourS extended arms and hands against a fixed surface.

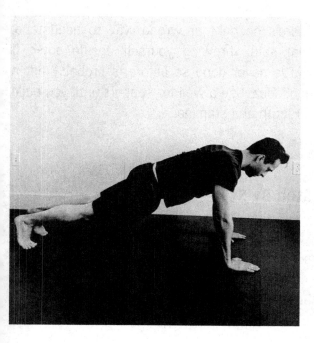

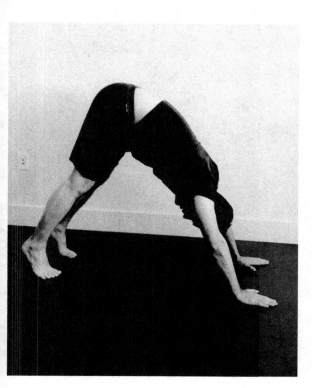

Let's look at that last sentence again. Does "doing a handstand" fit that definition? Yes, the arms are extended up over head (though the body is inverted) and the hands are against a fixed surface (the ground); the weight of the body is supported by the extended arms and hands. But that's not the only way to do it.

A standard plank (the "high plank" with arms extended) is also an example of handstanding. You support the weight of the body between the hands and the toes.

Another example is the wall-supported Standing Downward Dog. It's a very light example of handstanding, but it does count. (The classic Downward Dog is also an example of handstanding).

"Doing a handstand" has to look a certain way. Handstanding looks however you do it.

With that in mind, I'm not going to tell you how to handstand. This one is fully on you. You're going to have to take everything you have learned elsewhere in this program and apply it to this. Handstanding is your opportunity to grow and to prove to yourself that you understand your body and how it works.

What have you learned from the punches and rows that would help you stand on your hands?

What have you learned from the overhead stretch?

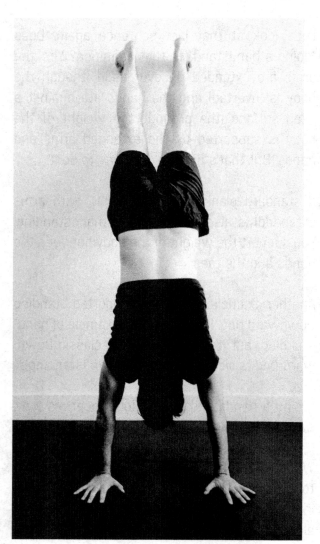

There's no right or wrong way to handstand. That said, throwing yourself upside down if you've never done so before is probably not a good idea. Use a wall for support until you build strength and stamina.

Step By Step

Step 1: Extend your arms and hands against a surface and support your bodyweight.

Step 2: Practice every day.

Movement Information

Movement Name
Handstanding

Difficulty
Level 4

Where you'll see it
Gymnastics
Martial arts
Breakdancing
Capoeira

What it Wakes Up
The entire body, especially the upper body.

Contraindications and Cautions
Compound exercises are more intense than the other movements in this sequence. Be sure you have cleared with your doctor that you're ready for advanced levels of exercise and exertion.

Don't do this movement if you have any kind of medical situation that can be negatively impacted from increased blood pressure. When you stand upside down, the blood pressure in the head increases dramatically, and it can take time for your body to adjust. Build up tolerance by practicing for weeks at a time.

Don't do this movement if you're pregnant.

You should also not do this movement if you have any issues with your shoulders, neck, or wrists.

If not performed carefully this can be a dangerous movement, causing damage to the

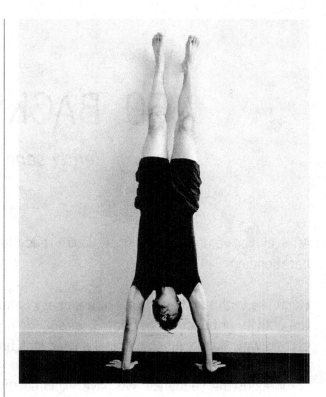

neck and spine. Move slowly and intentionally at all times, keeping the head stable.

If you have any type of neck pain or injury, do not perform this movement without the supervision and permission of a doctor.

Deepen the Movement
The more of your body that is inverted directly above the hands, the deeper the movement will become. A perfect handstand has 100% of the body above the hands.

In the Beginning...
Use a wall to support yourself until you are strong enough to support your weight.

Additional Research
Search: "How to do a handstand"

50. BACKBENDING

Gently bend backwards.

After all you've done to get here, you're ready for the final movement in the TheraQi sequence-backbending.

Much like with handstanding, I intentionally name this activity "backbending" to distinguish it as the activity of bending backwards, versus "doing a backbend." "Doing a backbend" has to look a certain way. Backbending can and should look however you feel comfortable.

Throughout the sequence, we have explored the idea of balance. Butterfly Stroke has Reverse Butterfly Stroke. Pushes have Pulls. In that spirit, Backbending is an important counter balance to all the bending we have been doing earlier. Additionally, the Hula movements have a habit of flattening the spine, and Backbending helps to restore the natural arch of the back. This is an important skill for you to have in your movement toolkit.

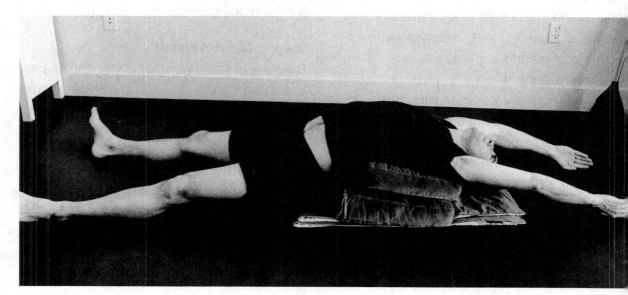

Also like with Handstanding, I'm not going to tell you how to backbend. Only you know what's right for you and your body. Explore. Experiment. Read up and research. Hire a coach, trainer or instructor. Go to a yoga class. But it also doesn't have to be that complicated. Buying one of those big Swiss exercise balls and leaning back on it is probably as effective a form of Backbending that you'll ever need. Don't make it harder than it needs to be. My favorite way to backbend is to lean back on my bed, and then slowly slide down onto the floor, using my mattress to support and bend my spine backward. Experiment with what works for you.

Step By Step

Only Step: Bend backward in a safe, sustainable, secure, and comfortable manner of your choosing.

MOVEMENT INFORMATION

Movement Name
Backbending

Difficulty
Level 3

Where you'll see it
Yoga
Dance
Martial arts

What it Wakes Up
Spine and lower back

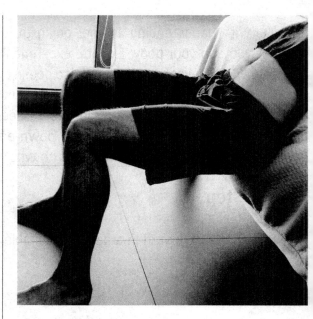

Contraindications and Cautions
Backbends are more intense than the other movements in this sequence, and as a spine specific movement, you must advance into this movement carefully. Be sure you have cleared with your doctor that you're ready for advanced levels of exercise and exertion. Always move slowly and in a controlled manner. Take your back seriously.

If not performed carefully this can be a dangerous movement, causing damage to the neck and spine. Move slowly and intentionally at all times, keeping the head stable.

If you have any type of neck pain or injury, do not perform this movement without the supervision and permission of a doctor.

Move slowly. At no time should you feel any pain or discomfort.

Do not over-extend.

Deepen the Movement
Keep practicing.

In the Beginning...
Use props to support yourself. Don't be a hero and try to "do" a perfect backbend without support. Use whatever props you can find to support your back, whether it's as casual as a pile of pillows, or as studied as a Swiss exercise ball.

Additional Research
Search: "Backbend" or "Yoga Backbend"

Becoming a TheraQi Instructor

I wrote this book out of a commitment to making healing movement accessible and enjoyable to anyone, regardless of age, body type, or fitness level. My vision is a world where people spend 30 minutes a day moving for the sheer pleasure of it, not because they have to, but because they want to. I see a world where everyone can be included in fitness, not just the people who are already fit. No more guilt, no more shame, no more inertia, no more excuses. When movement feels good, it happens naturally.

To make this world a reality, I'm on a mission to educate humanity about the benefits of gentle, dynamic flexibility exercises practiced as a daily routine. I want to reach as many people as possible. Research shows that only 3% of Americans are exercising every day. I'm out to change that, but I can't do it alone. I'm committed to creating a huge network of instructors that will impact their local communities by teaching the TheraQi method and the benefits it provides.

If you see the value in the TheraQi method and you can see the difference it would make for your family, friends, and community, please contact us to learn where and how you can become a licensed TheraQi instructor.

To purchase video training, to find a certified TheraQi instructor, or to become a certified TheraQi instructor yourself, visit our website.

www.theraqi.com

You may also follow us on social media.

fb.com/theraqi

twitter.com/theraqi

For bulk orders of this book, please call +1-212-666-4400

ABOUT THE AUTHOR

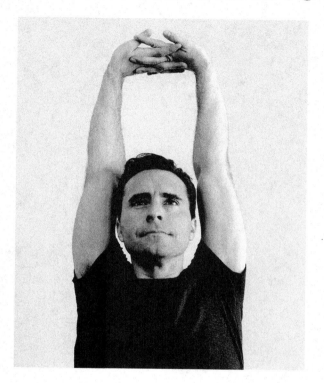

Jason Rockwood is a life-long movement enthusiast and the creator of the TheraQi movement method. An unabashed fan of self-help and personal development methodologies, Jason has dedicated his life to helping people be happy, healthy, and enlightened. Professionally, he has had a career in marketing and technology, where he championed the value of community and connection to help brands become more human-centered.

Jason developed the TheraQi movement method after traditional fitness methods failed him. The method is based on a decade-long study of kinesiology, martial arts, physical therapy and dance. This book is a natural outcome of his commitment to making complex wellness information accessible and achievable.

Jason earned a Bachelor of Arts in Communication from the University of Illinois at Urbana-Champaign and a Master of Science in Comparative Media Studies from the Massachusetts Institute of Technology. A native of Illinois, he now lives in Miami, Florida.

CPSIA information can be obtained
at www.ICGtesting.com
Printed in the USA
FSOW03n1038030118
43007FS